# A Poet's Recipe to Vegan Eating

**Published and distributed in the United States by**: Belle Publishing LLC
**www.bellepublishingllc.co**

**Cover and interior design**

**Belle Publishing LLC**



**Paperback ISBN: 13: 978-1-7337063-3-9**

**eBook ISBN:**

**10 9 8 7 6 5 4 3 2 1**

**First Edition**

**January 2020**

PRINTED IN THE UNITED STATES OF AMERICA

# A Poet's Recipe to Going Vegan

Simple, Easy and Delicious Vegan/Plant-Based Meals.

# Table of contents

06 Entrees

62 Desserts

82 Smoothies

120 Handy Tips

125 Index

128 Acknowledgments

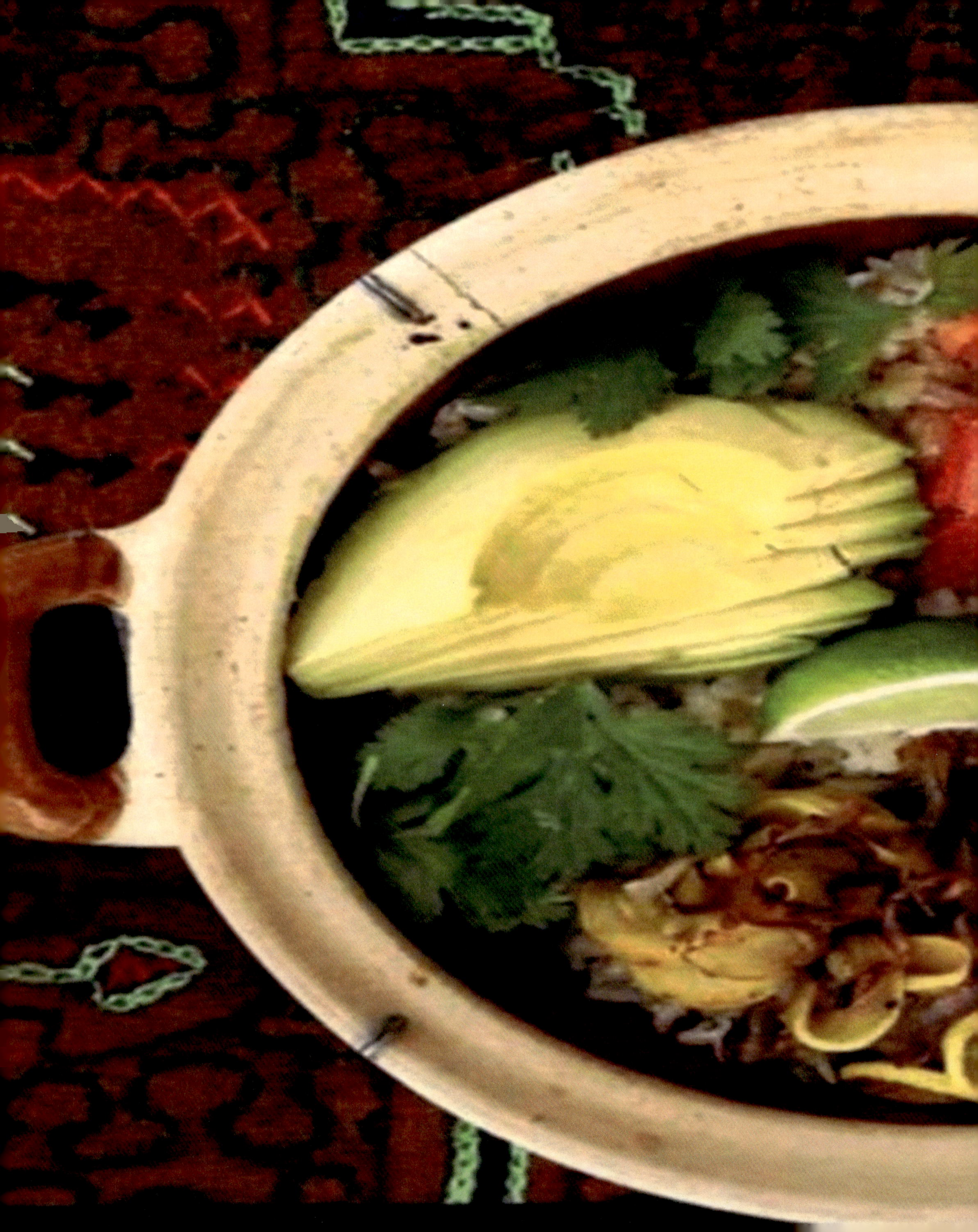

# ENTREES

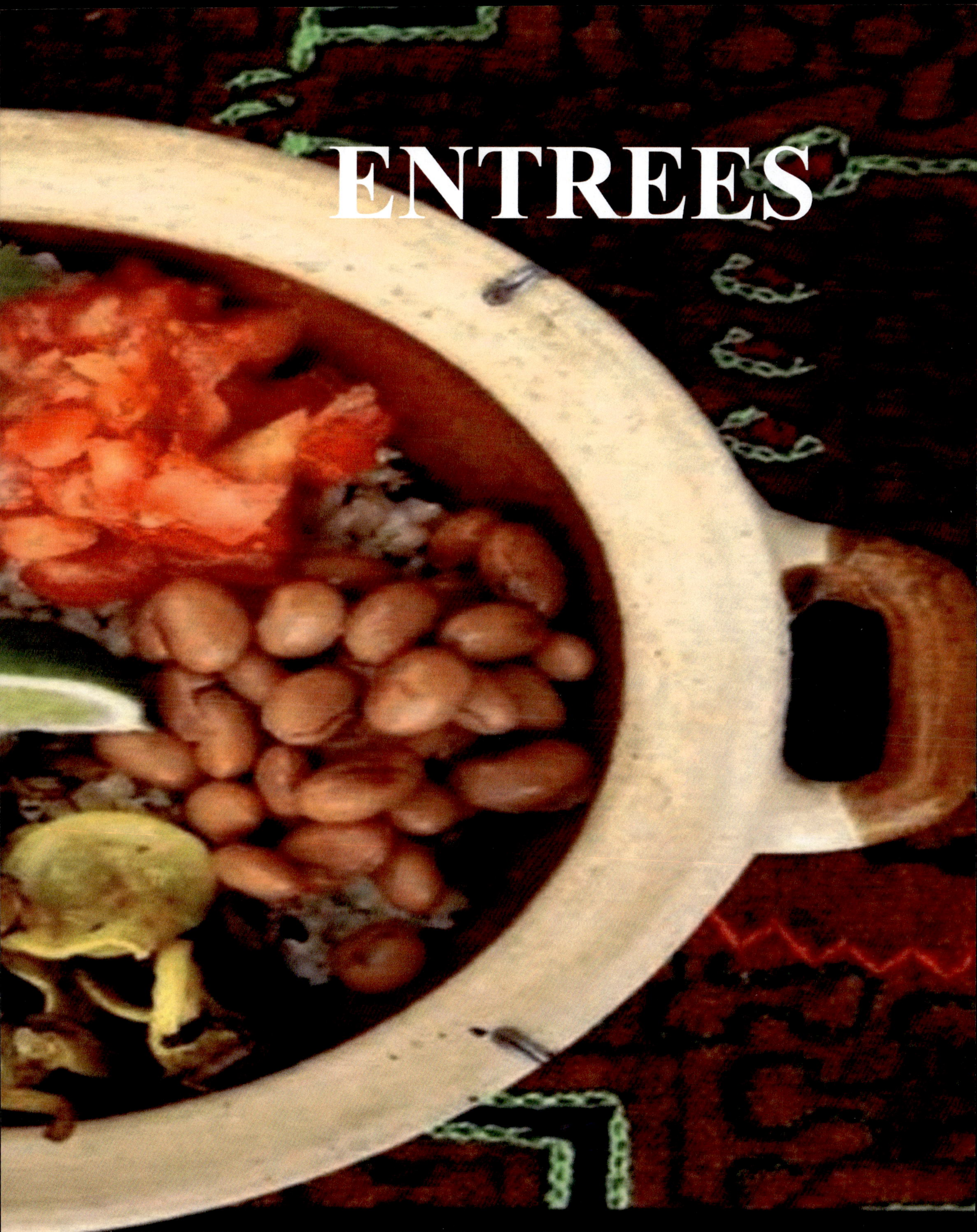

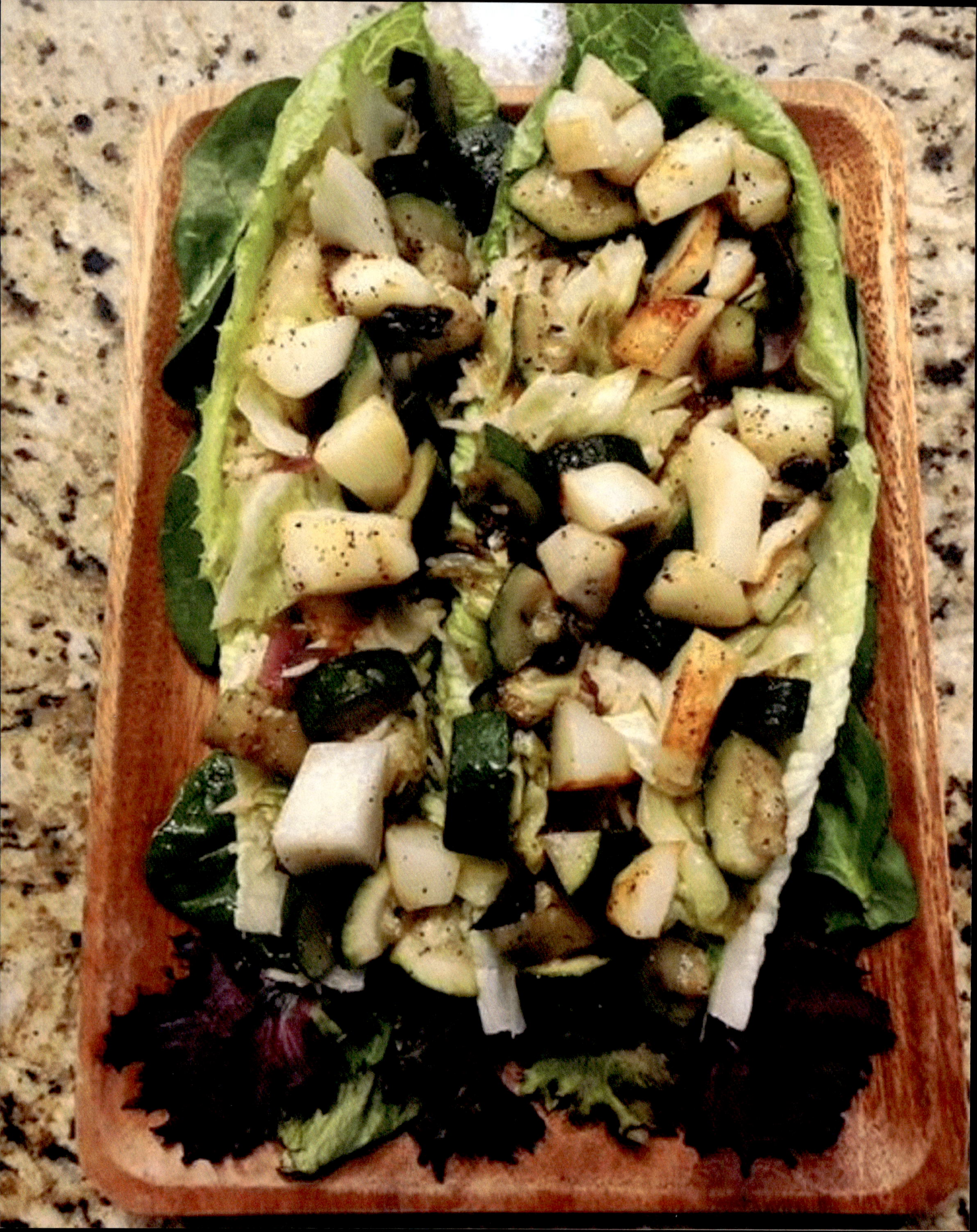

# Vegan Stuffed Romaine Lettuce

**Ingredients:**

2 romaine lettuce stalks

1 cup zucchini, diced

1cup potatoes, diced

1/2 red onions, chopped

2 cup cabbage, chopped

1 cup basmati rice

1 tsp Himalayan salt & 1 tsp pepper

2 tbsp grapeseed oil

**Directions:**

Heat the oil in a skillet. Add the potatoes, red onions, cabbage, zucchini, salt and pepper. Cook for 10-15 minutes.

Cook basmati rice according to package.

Spoon the basmati rice on top of the romaine lettuce.

Add the sautéed veggie on top of the basmati rice.

Eat and Enjoy all your veggies at one time

**Preparation time:15 minutes**
**Total time:25 minutes**
**Makes:2 servings**

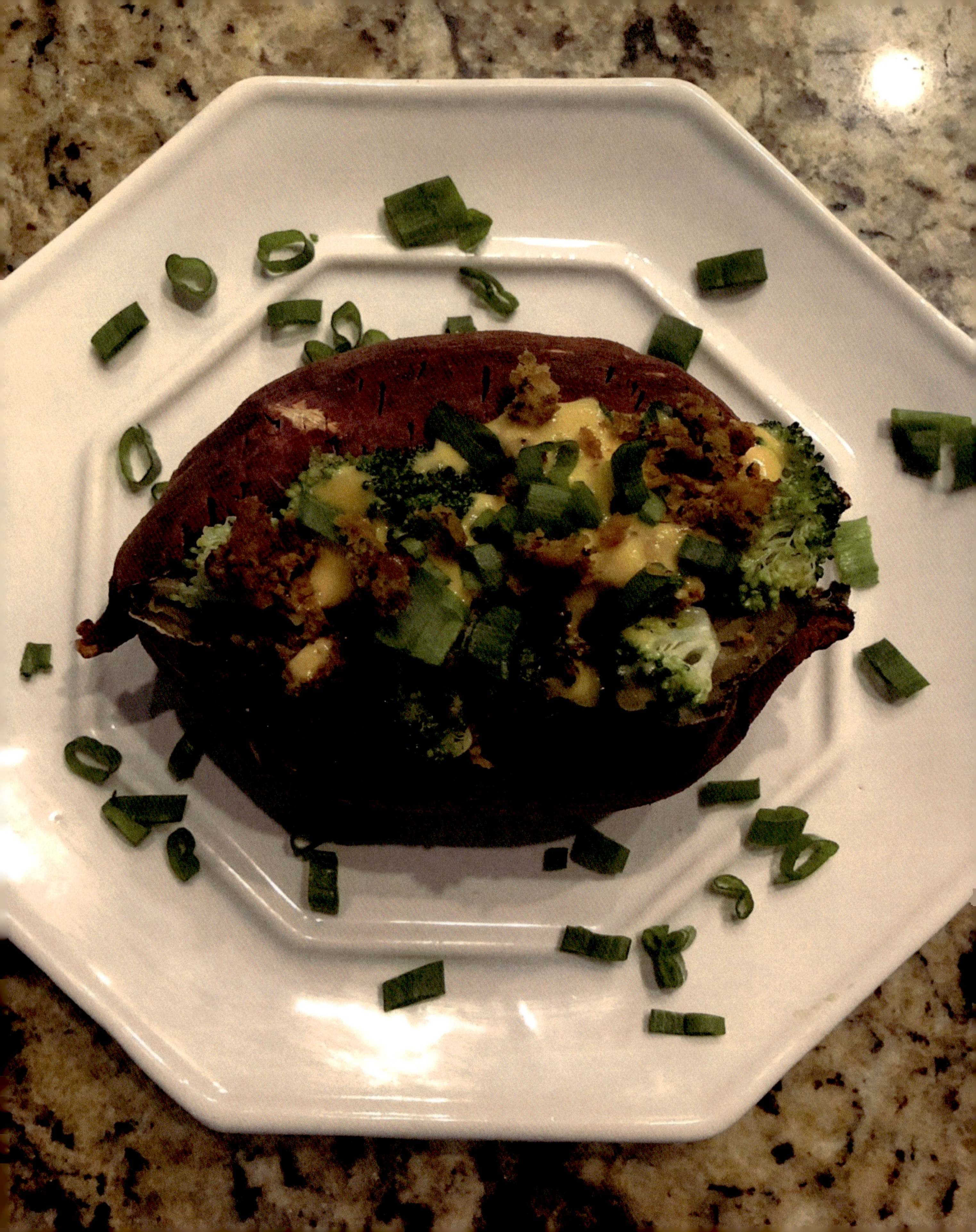

# Vegan Stuffed Japanese Sweet Potato

**Ingredients:**

2 Japanese sweet potatoes

4 falafel balls

1 1/2 broccoli, diced

3/4 green onions, chopped

1/2 cup cheese (your choice)

1/2 almond milk (your choice of non-dairy milk)

2 tbsp. grapeseed oil

**Directions:**

Pre-heat the oven to 350°F

Bake Japanese sweet potato for 45-60 minutes.

In a small pan add almond milk and vegan cheese cook for 3-5 minutes.

Heat the oil in a skillet. Add the falafel balls, broccoli, and cook for 8-10 minutes.

Spoon the falafel balls and broccoli on to the Japanese sweet potato.

Add the melted vegan cheese on top of the potato.

Add the chopped green onions.

Enjoy your all-in stuffed potato

**Preparation time:25**
**Total time:45 minutes**
**Makes:2 servings**

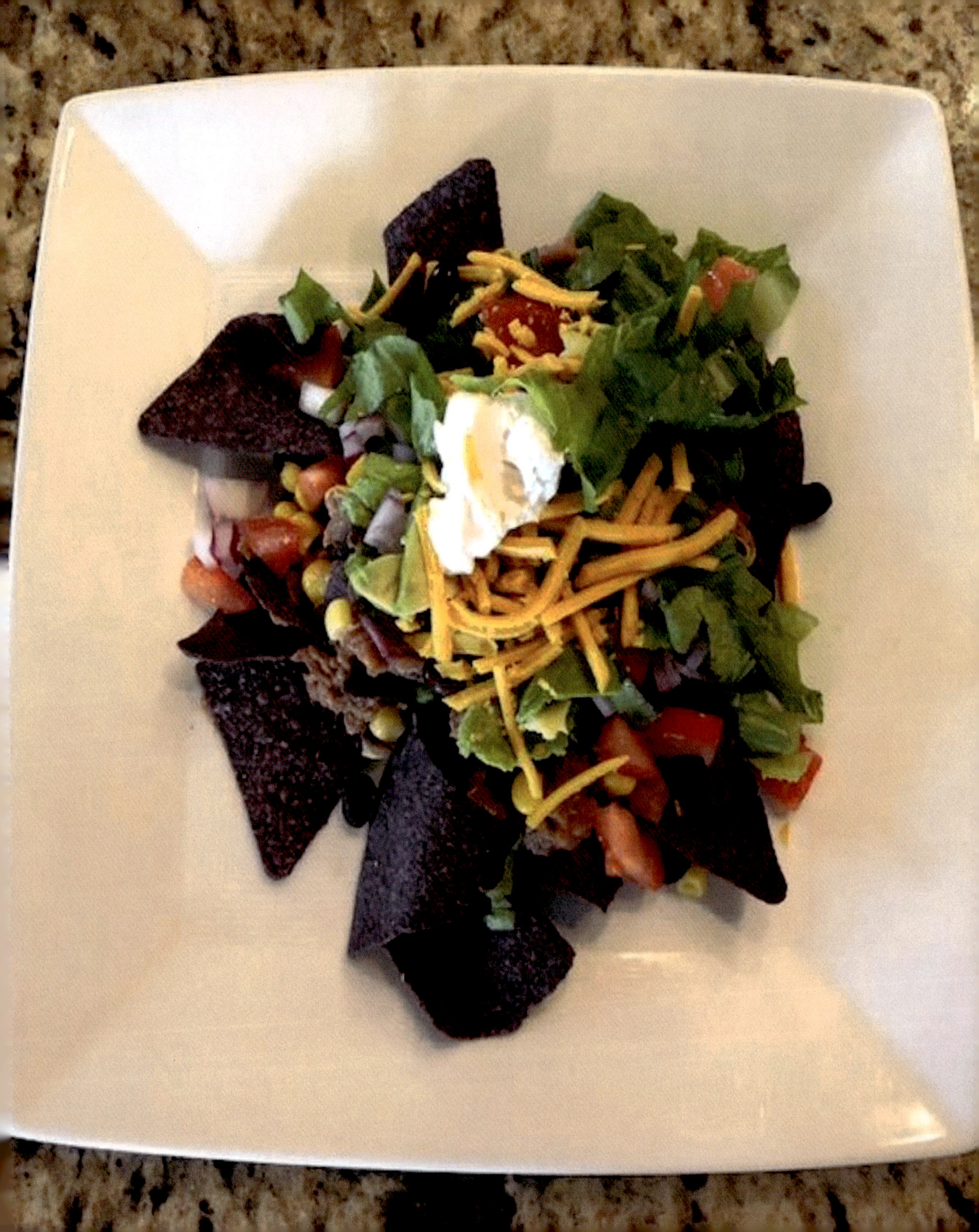

# Vegan Loaded Nachos

**Ingredients:**

1/2 can refried brown beans

1/2 can black beans

1 handful organic blue corn chips

1/2 cup organic kernel corn

1/2 cup romaine lettuce (chopped)

1/2 cup organic tomatoes (diced)

1/2 cup organic red onion (diced)

1/2 cup shredded cheddar vegan cheese (your choice)

1 tbsp vegan sour cream

1 tbsp of grapeseed oil

**Directions**

In a small skillet heat the grapeseed oil. Add the refried beans cook for 5-8 minutes.

In a small pan heat the black beans for 5-8 minutes.

On a medium plate add chips, refried beans, black beans, romaine lettuce, corn, tomatoes, red onion, shredded cheese, and sour cream.

One bite at a time! Enjoy

**Preparation time:15 minutes**
**Total time:20 minutes**
**Makes:4 servings**

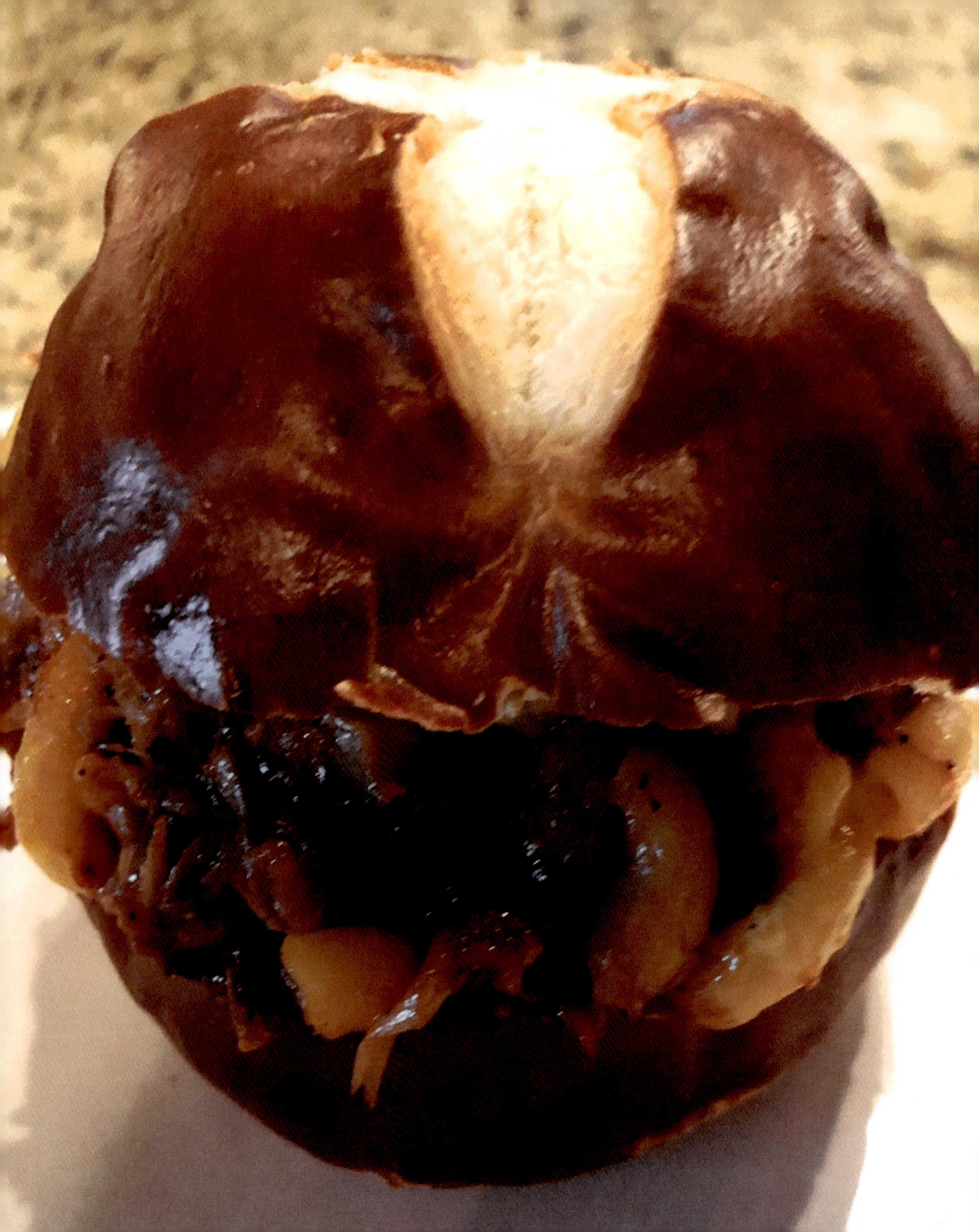

# Mac & Cheese Barbecue Sandwich

**Ingredients:**

1 16 oz can jack fruit (Trader Joe's Brand)

1 cup barbecue sauce (your choice)

Pretzilla Bun (your choice)

1 cup vegan Shredded cheddar cheese (Daiya shredded cheddar cheese)

1/2 cup grated parmesan cheese (Vegan Go Veggie)

1 tbsp vegan sour cream (Tofutti milk free)

1 cup elbow macaroni (Tolerant Simply Legumes Green Lentil Pasta) cook according to package

1/2 tsp Himalayan salt & pepper

1/2 tsp Garlic powder

1/2 tsp Onion powder

¼ cup almond milk

2 tbsp grapeseed oil

**Directions:**

Pre-heat the oven to 350° degrees.

Heat the oil in a medium skillet. Add the shredded jack fruit, Himalayan salt, pepper, garlic powder, onion powder, cook for 7-10 minutes. Add barbecue sauce.

In a medium pan cook the elbow macaroni. Drain the macaroni. Add the shredded cheese, parmesan cheese, sour cream, almond milk; combine well and cook 5-8 minutes.

In a medium baking dish add the cook barbecue jack fruit spread evenly. Add the cook mac & cheese on top spread evenly. Bake for 10-15 minutes.

Add a couple of spoonfuls of the mac & cheese barbecue dish on the Pretzilla bun.

Enjoy!

**Preparation time:20 minutes**
**Total time:35 minutes**
**Makes:4 servings**

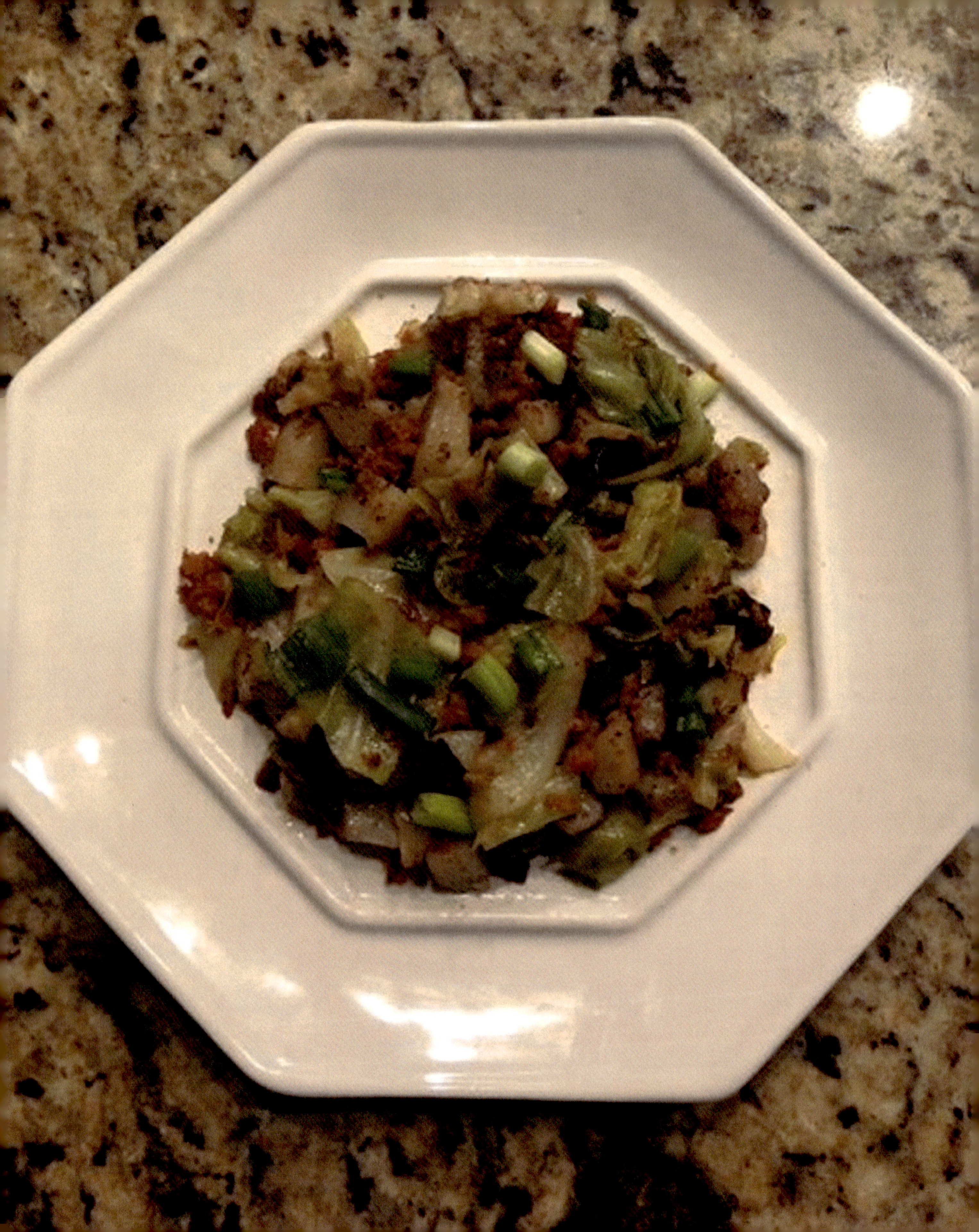

# Vegan Cabbage Potato Hash

**Ingredients:**

Small or medium cabbage (red cabbage optional)

4 medium potatoes

1/2 red onion (chopped roughly)

2 Beyond meat patties (your choice)

3/4 cup green onions

2 cloves garlic

1 1/2 tbsp. grape seed oil

1 tsp Himalayan salt

1 tsp black pepper

2 tbsp. nutritional yeast (optional)

**Directions:**

Heat the oil in a large skillet. Add the potatoes, cabbage, red onions, and 1 chopped garlic, and sauté the vegetables for 5-8 minutes, or until the vegetables have softened.

Add Himalayan salt, pepper, nutritional yeast.

Heat the oil in a small skillet. Add the two Beyond Meat Patties. Add Himalayan salt, pepper, 1 chopped garlic, nutritional yeast. Cook for 10-12 minutes, or until fully cooked.

Transfer ingredients to individual serving plates, and garnish with chopped green onions and serve. So delicious!

**Preparation time:15 minutes**
**Total time:30 minutes**
**Makes:3 servings**

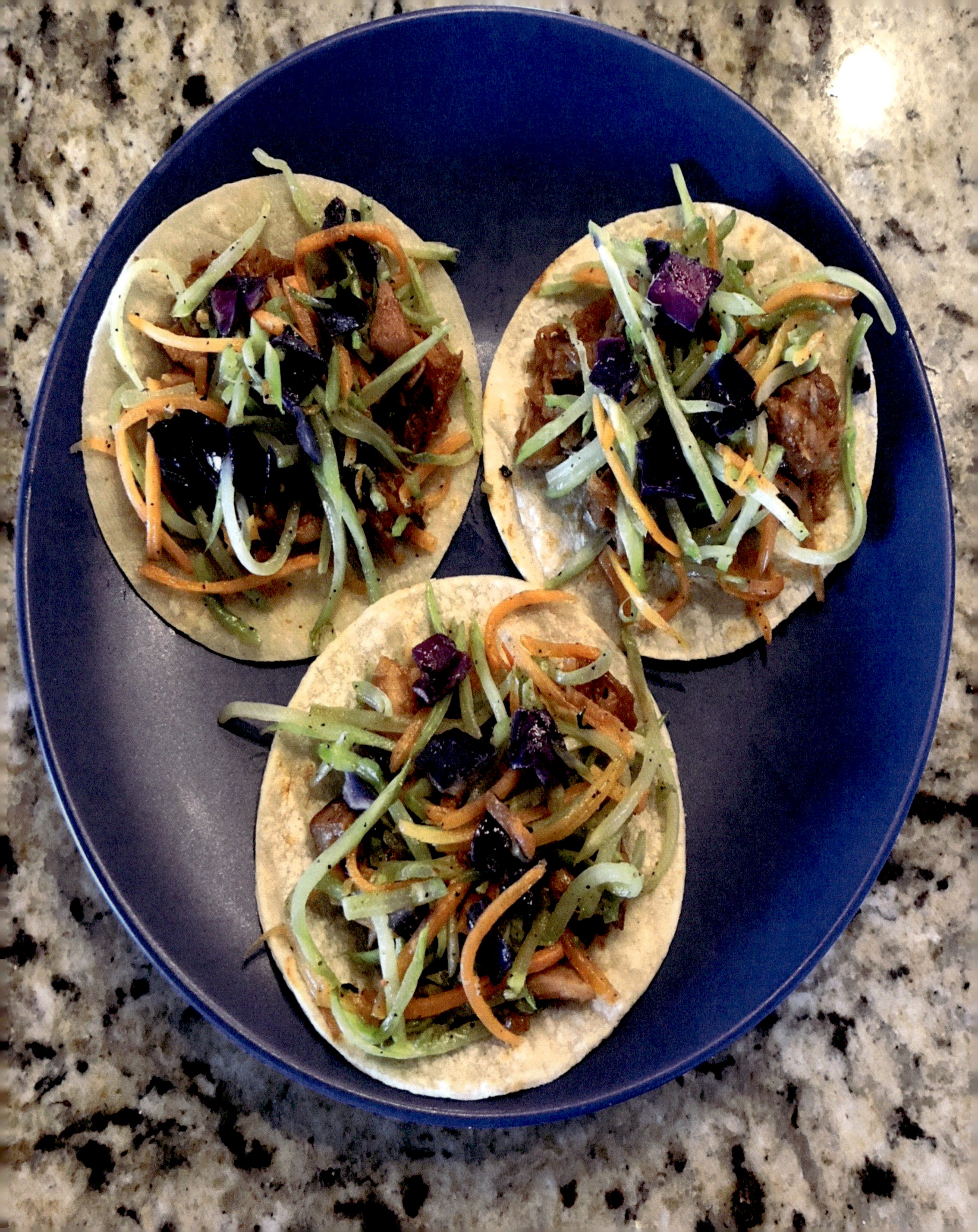

# Barbecue Street Tacos

**Ingredients:**

1 1/2 cup Broccoli coleslaw

1 can jackfruit in brine (dried and rinsed) (shredded the jackfruit)

1/2 cup barbecue sauce (your choice)

1 tsp Himalayan salt

1 tsp black pepper

1 tsp garlic powder

1 tsp onion powder

1 tbsp. grape seed oil

1 tbsp. liquid smoke

1 tbsp. amino

1 tsp nutritional yeast (optional)

6 mini fajita tortillas

**Directions:**

Heat the oil in a medium skilled. Add jackfruit, Himalayan salt, pepper, garlic powder, onion powder, and nutritional yeast, liquid smoke, and amino. Cook for 10-12 minutes, or until well cooked.

Heat the oil in a medium skilled. Add broccoli coleslaw, Himalayan salt, black pepper, and nutritional yeast. Cook for 8-10 minutes.

Remover broccoli slaw from skillet into medium bowl. Add mini fajita tortillas in skillet. Cook for 3-5 minutes on each side.

Place min fajita tortillas on small plate. Add cook jackfruit. add sautéed broccoli coleslaw and serve

**Preparation time:15 minutes**
**Total time:25 minutes**
**Makes:4 servings**

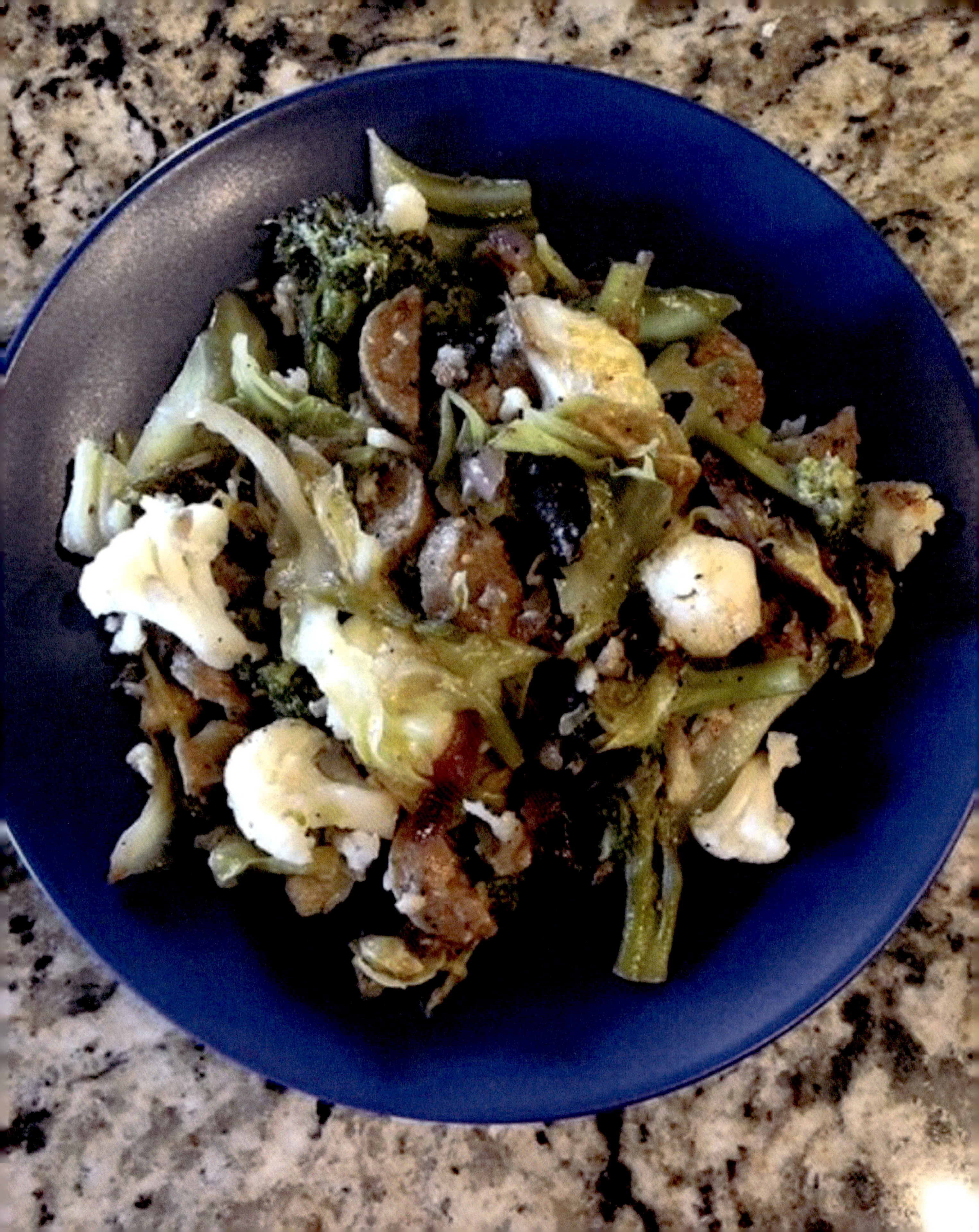

# Mixed Veggie Pan-Fry

**Ingredients:**

2 cups broccoli

2 cups cauliflower

1/2 cup red onion (sliced)

2 1/2 cabbage

1 cups portobello mushroom

2 Field Roast Apple sage sausage (cut pieces)

2 tbsp grape seed oil

1/2 cup organic low sodium vegetable broth

1 tsp Himalayan salt

1 tsp garlic powder

1 tsp black pepper

2 tsp nutritional yeast

**Directions:**

Heat the oil in a medium skillet. Add cabbage, cauliflower, broccoli, mushrooms, red onions, Himalayan salt, black pepper, garlic powder, nutritional yeast. Cook for 12-15 minutes.

Add sausage, vegetable broth. Steam for 10-12 minutes.

Spoon the sautéed vegetables onto a medium plate. Serve at once.

**Preparation time:10 minutes**
**Total time:20 minutes**
**Makes:4 servings**

***I Can and I Will***

*Who said my dreams were only on paper.*

*I manifest what I want in life.*

*I can and I will be H.H.W.*

*Happy, healthy and wealthy, in that order.*

*Just because your dreams sat on paper and the ink has faded away, now you can't even see what was meant to be.*

*There is so much power in knowing you Can and Will, because people really wouldn't understand that thoughts activate reality.*

*My beliefs in my dreams will continue to align and show through my actions to give you inspiration in your I CAN, and I WILL.*

*I Can and I will*

***Poetically Vegan***

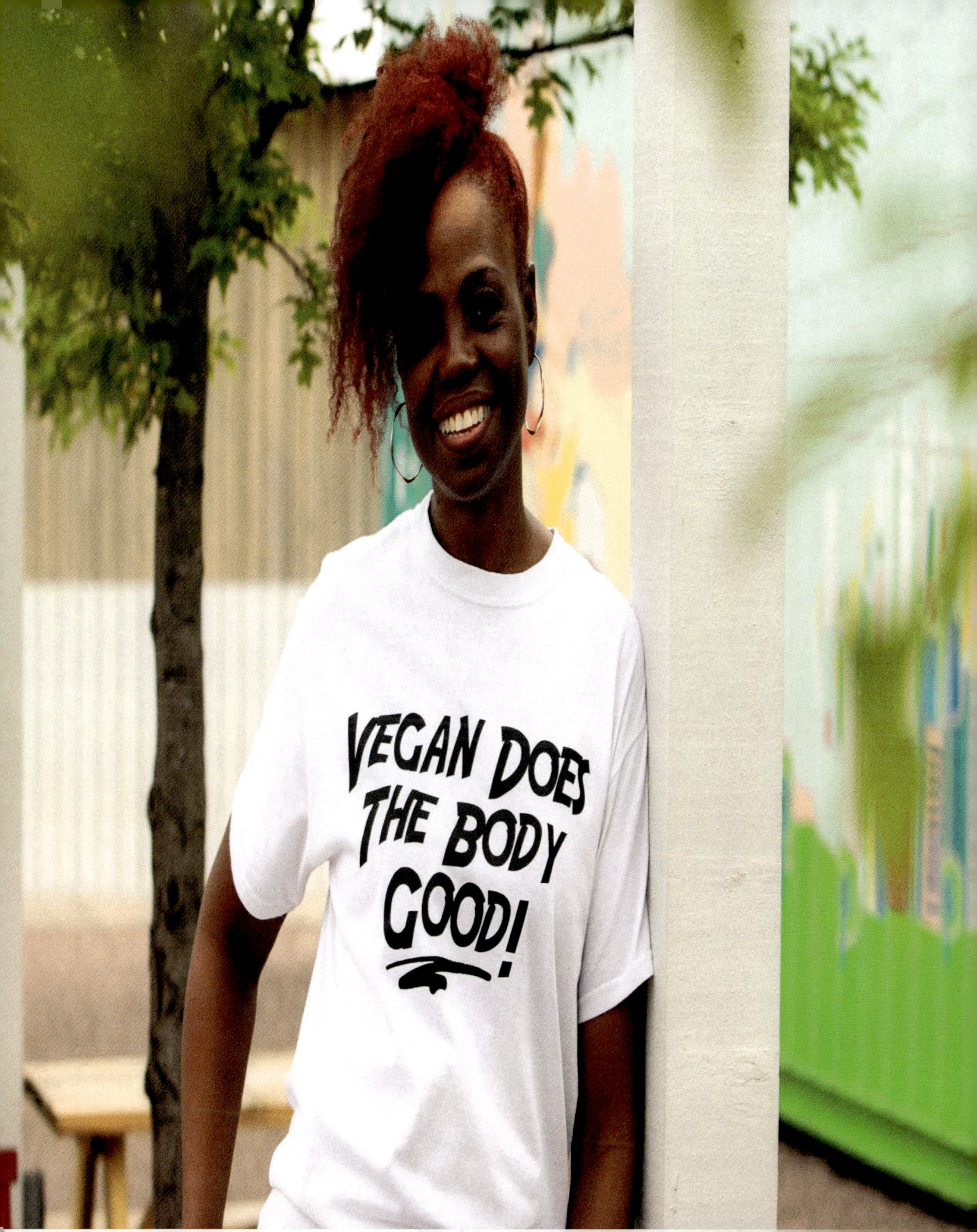
VEGAN DOES
THE BODY
GOOD!

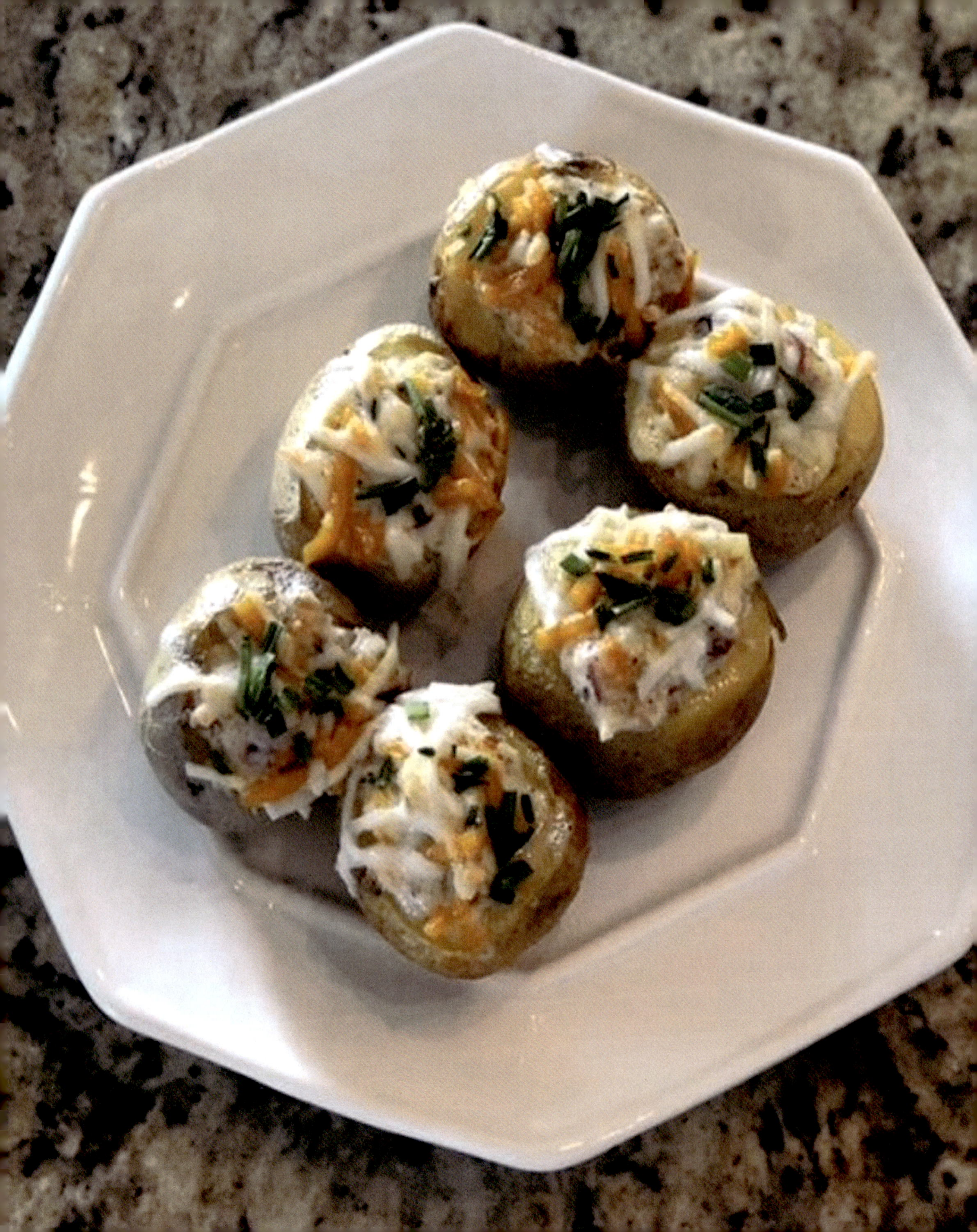

# Vegan Double Baked Yukon Potatoes

**Ingredients:**

6 small Yukon potatoes

1/2 cup Daiya cheddar style shredded cheese

1/2 cup Daiya mozzarella cheese

3/4 cup red onion (chop finely)

3/4 cup green onion (chop finely)

2 tbsp Tofutti vegan sour cream (your choice)

2 tbsp melted vegan butter

3/4 cup almond milk

1/2 tsp Himalayan salt

1/2 tsp black pepper

**Directions:**

Pre-heat the oven to 325°F

Place potatoes on a baking sheet. Bake for 20-35 minutes, or until tender.

Take potatoes out of the oven and let cool for 5-10 minutes.

In a medium bowl, scoop the potato meat. Add Himalayan salt, pepper, garlic powder, red onion, sour cream, almond milk, and cheese.

Spoon the mixture into the potatoes and top with more cheese. Add melted vegan butter. Bake for 10-15 minutes.

Place the potatoes on a medium dish. Garnish with green onions and serve

**Preparation time:15 minutes**
**Total time:35 minutes**

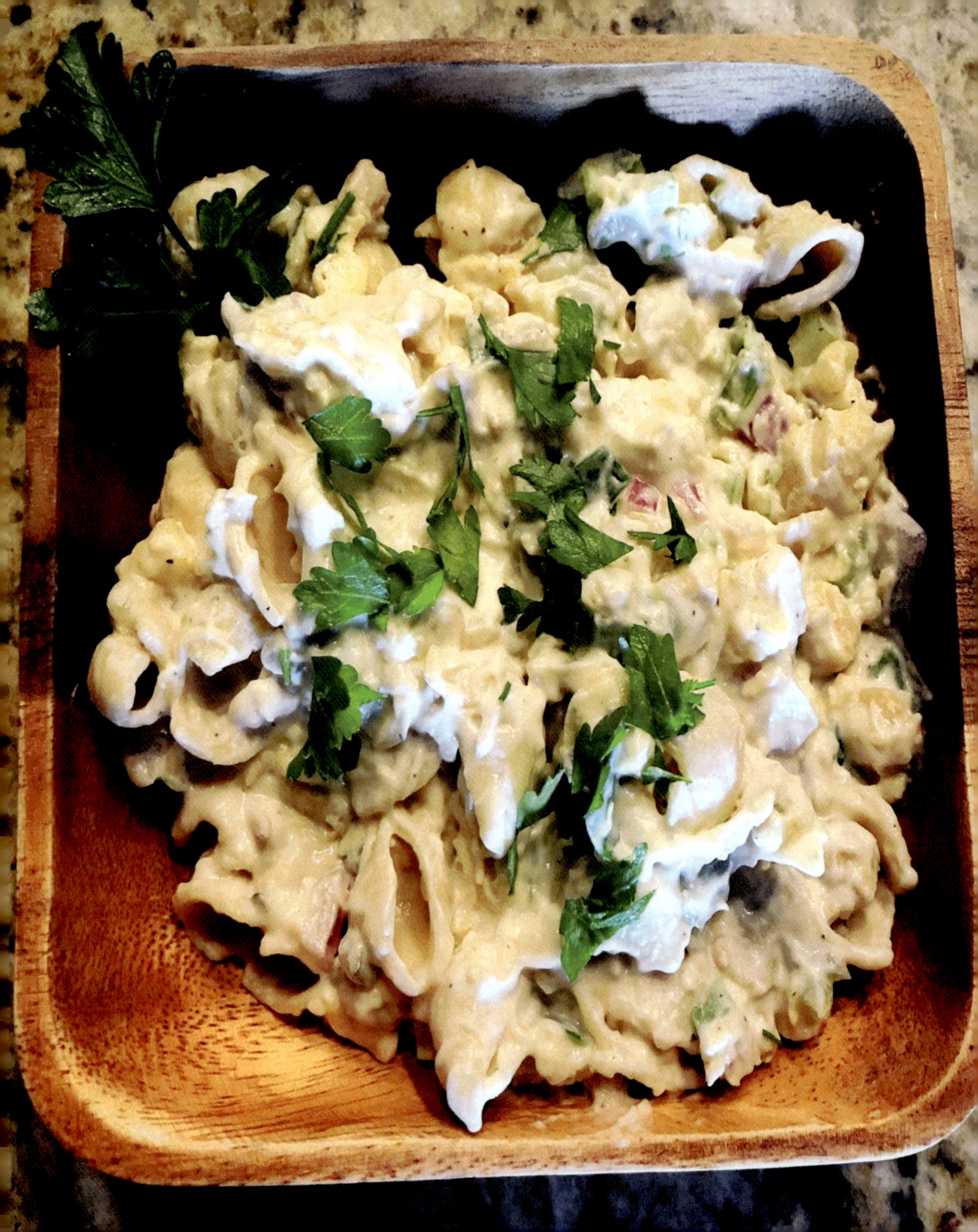

# Vegan Chickpea Macaroni Chipotle Salad/Sandwich

**Ingredients:**

Chickpeas 1 can (14-16 oz), drain & risen off, remove the outer skin of the chickpea, put in food processor for 30 seconds or use a folk.
Chickpea shell macaroni (cook as directed on package).
3/4 cup celery (chopped)
1/2 cup red onions (chopped)
1/2 cup green onions (chopped)
2 tbsp relish (dill or sweet)
3/4 cup vegan mayo (just mayo) or your choice
1/2 cup vegan chipotle mayo (just chipotle mayo) or your choice
1 tbsp nutritional yeast
1/2 cup vegan cheddar shredded cheese
1/2 cup vegan mozzarella cheese
2 tbsp vegan sour cream
1/2 tsp Himalayan salt & black pepper

**Directions:**

In a large bowl add chickpeas, shell macaroni, just mayo, chipotle mayo, relish, nutritional yeast (optional), salt & pepper, mix.
Next add celery, red onions, green onions, mix together until combined well.
Chill 40 minutes. Serve on a pretzel bun or crackers. Chill & Enjoy!

**Preparation time:15 minutes**
**Total time:30 minutes**
**Makes:4 servings**

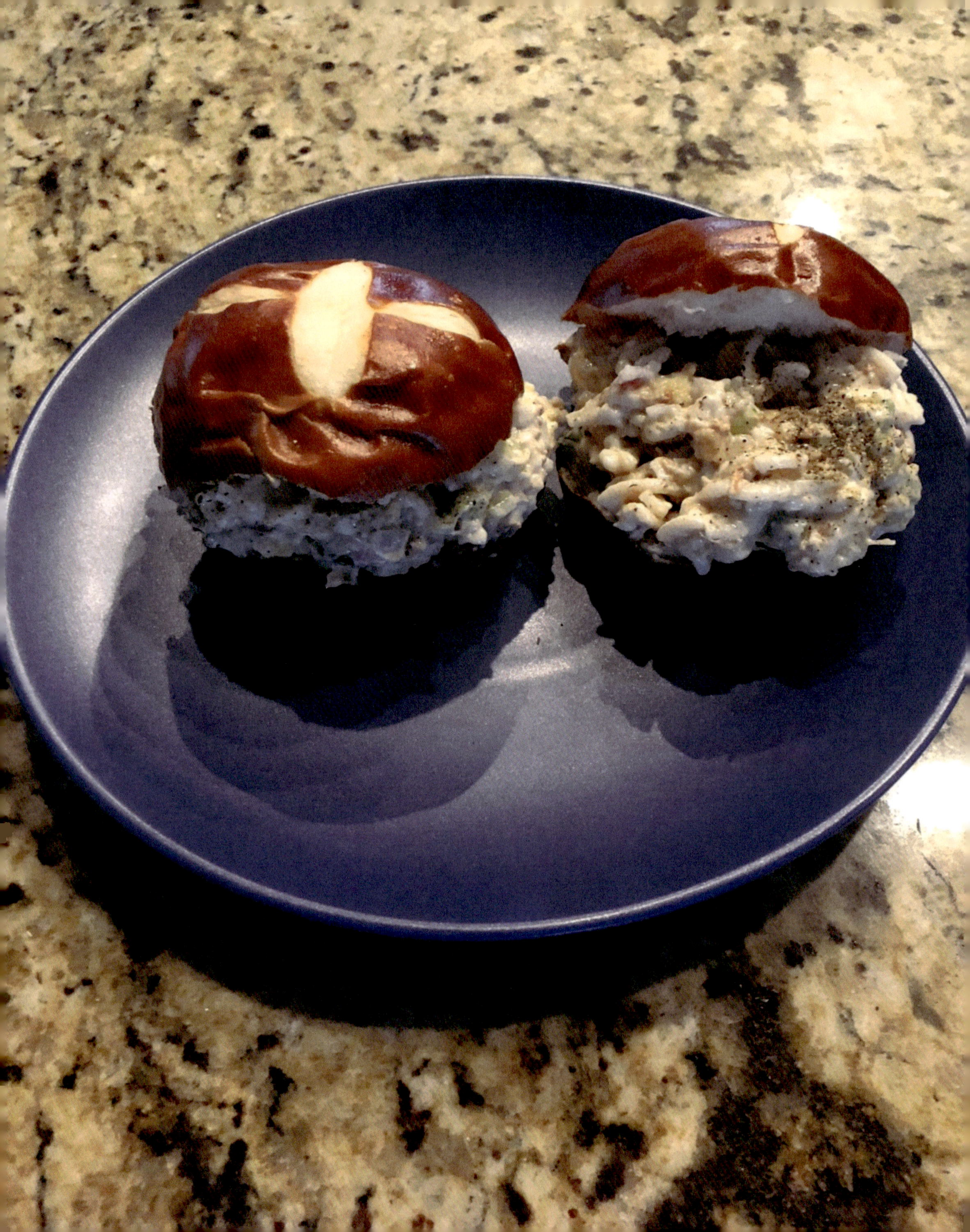

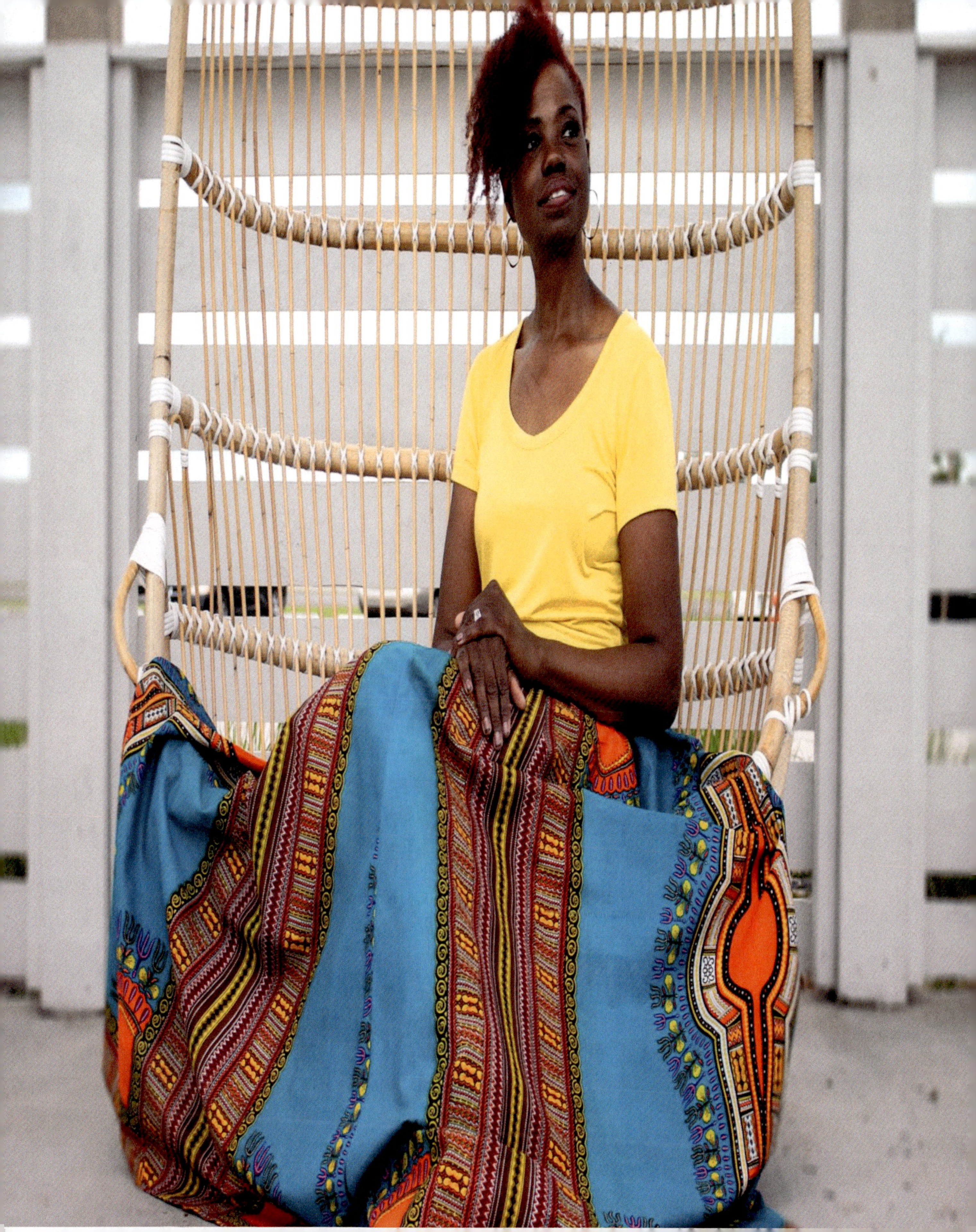

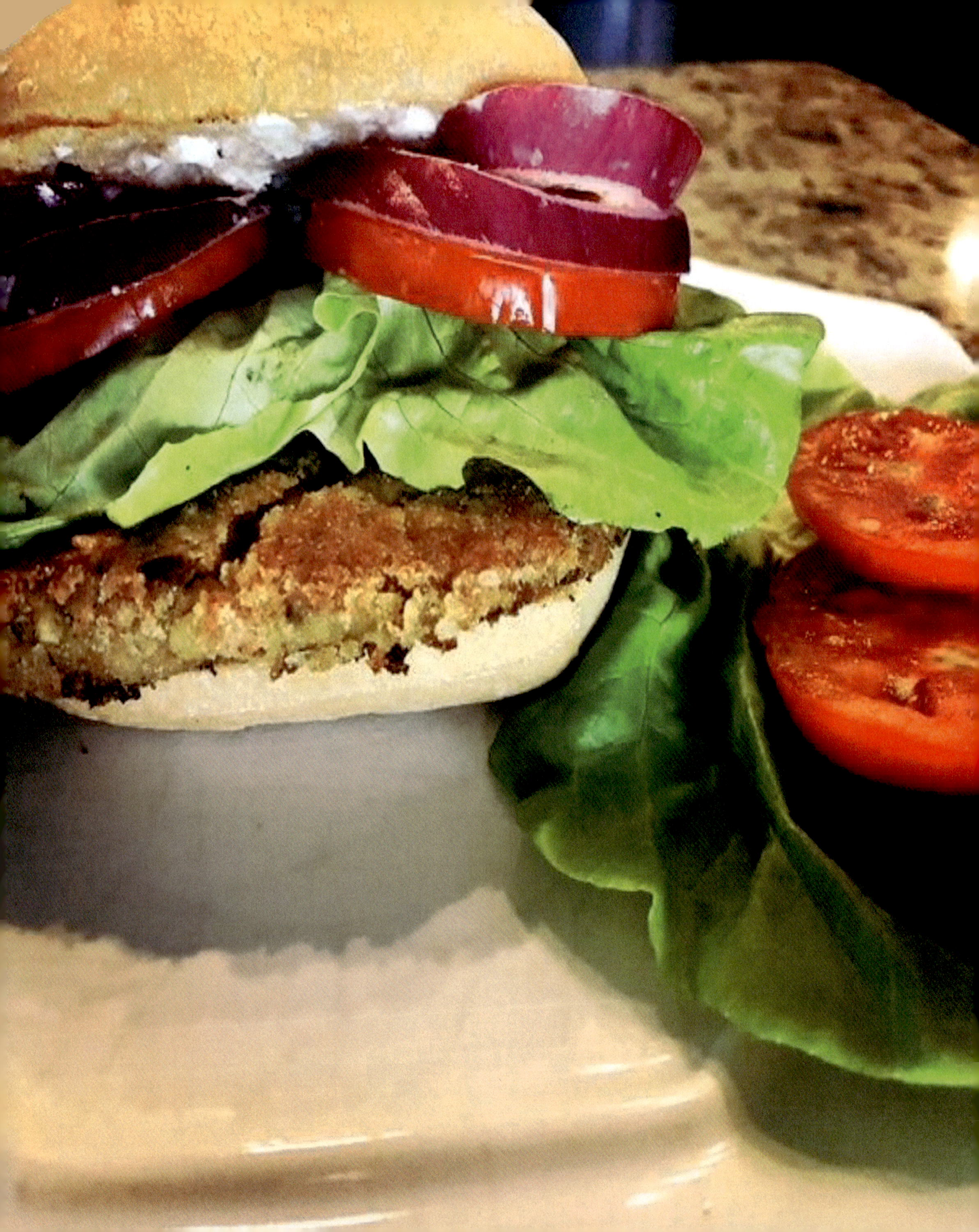

# Golden Brown Falafel Burger

**Ingredients:**

Golden brown falafel mixer (Pg33)

1/2 Red onions (sliced)

1 tomatoes (sliced)

8 leaves butterhead lettuce

1/2 tbsp vegan mayo (Just Mayo) or your choice

1/2 tbsp grapeseed oil

4 tbsp spelt flour

4 vegan buns (O'Doughs) or your choice

**Directions:**

Using lightly floured hands, form the mixture into 4 equal-sized burgers. Let chill in the refrigerator for 30 minutes.

Heat the oil in a small skillet. Cover the burger patties with the spelt flour, shaking off any excess. Cook the falafel burger for about 3-4 minutes on each side or until golden brown.

Remove the burger from the skillet onto a plate. Heat the buns in the same skillet for about 2-3 minutes. Transfer buns onto a plate. Add the vegan mayo on each side of the bun.

Place the cooked falafel burger on the bun. Add the butterhead lettuce leaves (**Cook's Tip:** Wash all produce to remove any dirt and pesticides), sliced tomatoes, and sliced red onions on top of cooked falafel burger.

Enjoy!

**Preparation time:20 minutes**
**Total time:30 minutes**
**Makes:8 servings**

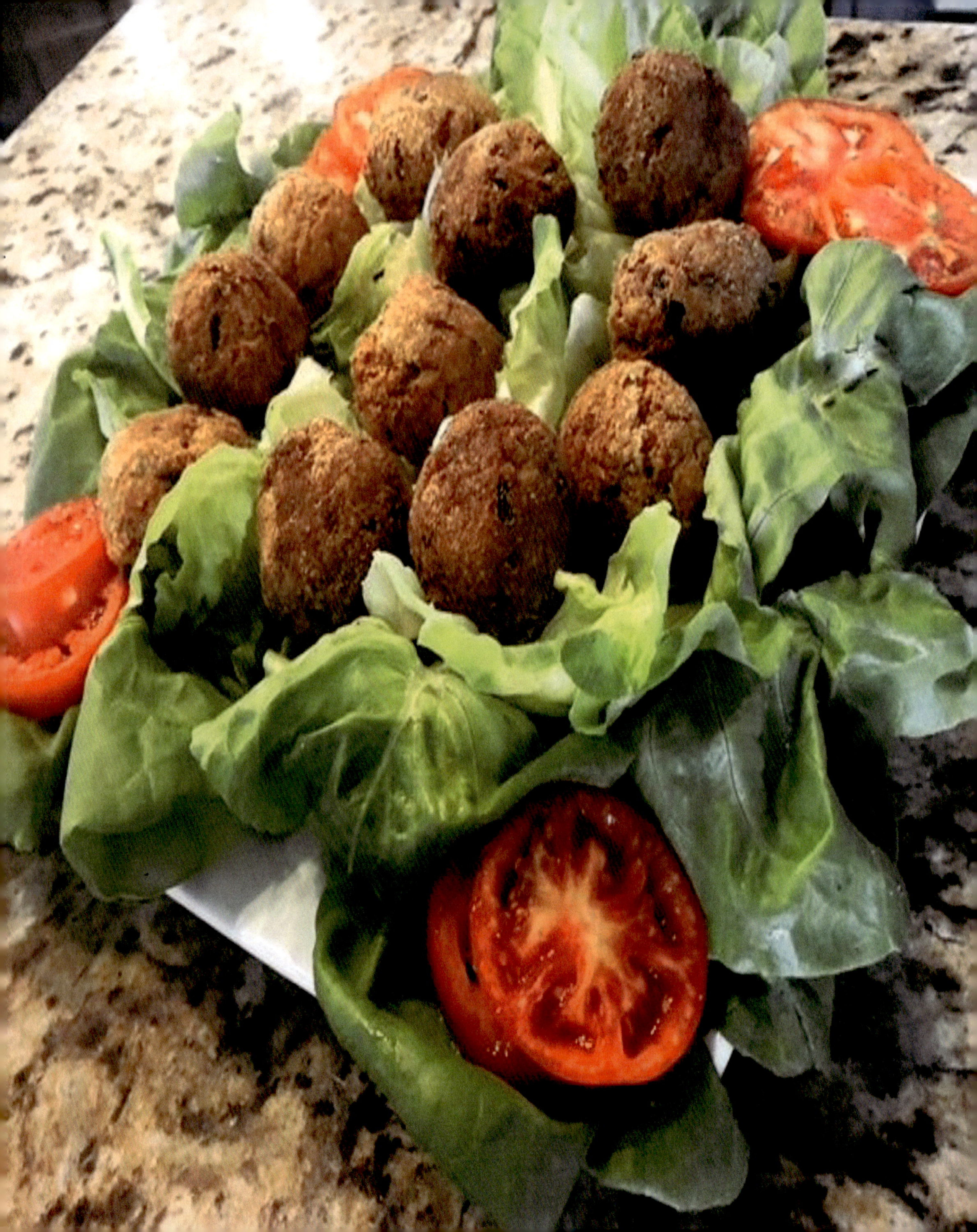

# Golden Brown Falafel Balls

**Ingredients:**

2 cans chickpeas

1/2 cup chickpea flour

1 cup red onion (chopped)

1/2 cup red bell pepper

1/2 cup green bell pepper

1 garlic clove (chopped)

2 tsp cumin

1 tsp coriander

1 tsp sage

1 tsp smoked paprika

½ tsp Himalayan salt

½ tsp black pepper

1 tbsp nutritional yeast (optional)

½ cup breadcrumbs

1 tbsp ground chia seeds

1 cup spelt flour

1 tbsp starch

½ tbsp avocado oil

1 ½ cup avocado oil (deep frying)

**Directions:**

In a medium-sized mixing bowl combine add the chickpeas and mash them with a potato masher. Stir in red onions, red bell pepper, green bell pepper, garlic until thoroughly combine.

Add the cumin, coriander, sage, smoke paprika, Himalayan salt, black pepper, nutritional yeast, breadcrumbs, chia seeds, starch, 1/2 tbsp avocado oil mix until thoroughly combine

Next in another medium-sized mixing bowl add the spelt flour. Shape the mix into walnut-size balls. Let chill in the refrigerator for 30 minutes. Roll the balls into the spelt flour, shaking off any excess.

Heat the oil for deep-frying in a large, heavy-bottom pan. Deep fry the falafel in batches for 3-4 minutes, or until golden brown.

Remove the falafel from the oil with a slotted spoon and dry on paper towels.

Serve with the Pearl Cous Cous salad (pg. 45) or your favorite sauce.

**Preparation time:20 minutes**
**Total time:25 minutes**
**Makes:4 servings**

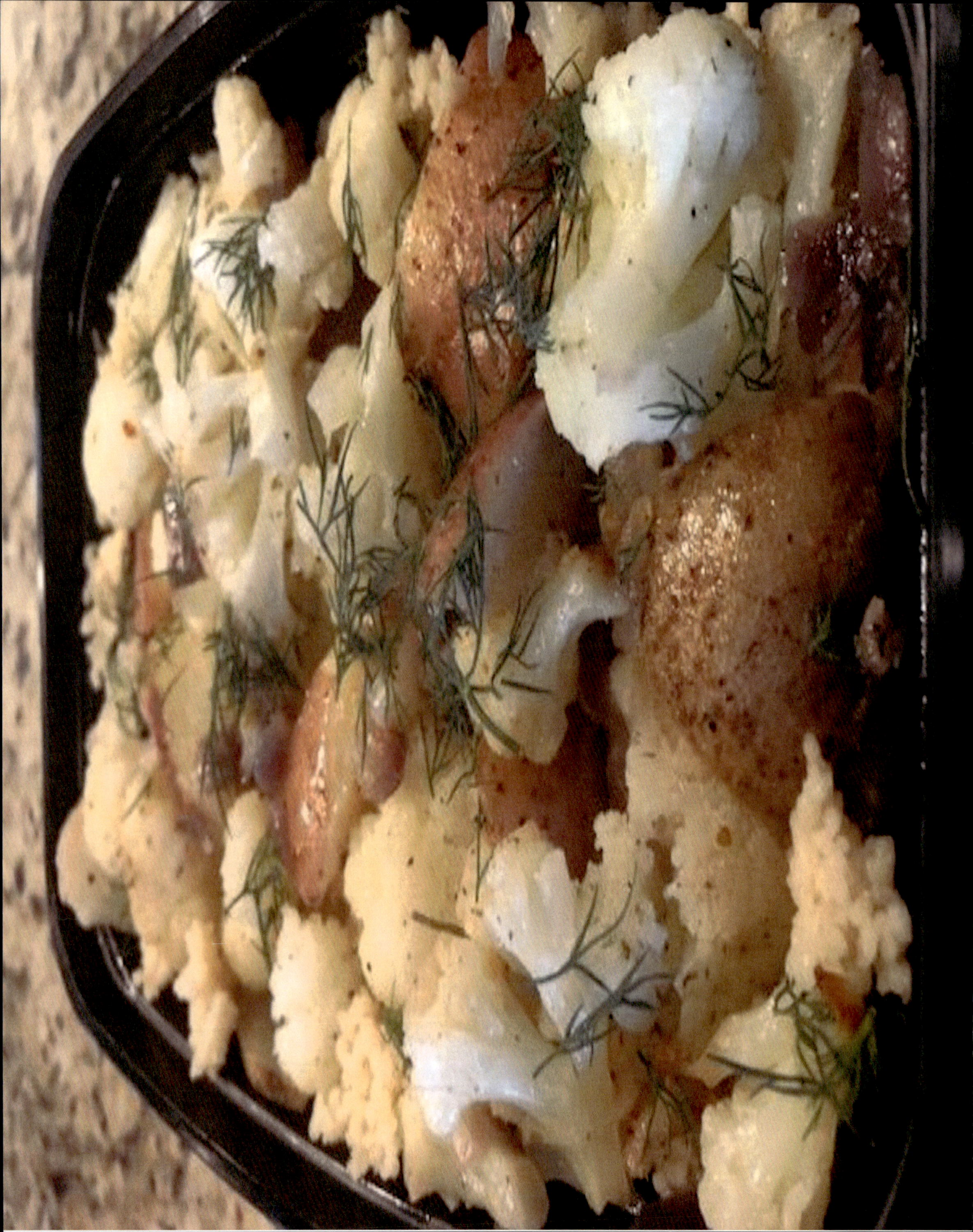

# Double Cauliflower Black Truffle

**Ingredients:**

1 medium Cauliflower (chopped)

4 small red potatoes (cut in quarters)

1/2 red onions (chopped)

1 1/2 cup cous cous (cook according to the package directions)

(**Cook's Tip:** Use a rice cooker for best results)

1 tsp black truffle salt

1/2 tsp Himalayan salt

1/2 tsp black pepper

1/2 tsp garlic powder

1/2 onion powder

2 tbsp avocado oil

2 tsp fresh dill (garnish)

Foil

**Directions:**

Pre-heat the oven to 350°F.

Place the chopped cauliflower, red potatoes, and red onions on a baking pan.

Add the oil, black truffle salt, and black pepper on top of the vegetables.

Cover with foil and bake for 25-30 minutes or until tender

Cook the couscous according to according to package directions. Add Himalayan salt, black pepper, garlic powder and onion powder to taste.

Transfer cous cous to serving plate. Place cooked vegetables on top of the cous cous. Garnish with fresh dill.

Serve and Enjoy.

**Preparation time:25 minutes**
**Total time:20 minutes**
**Makes: 4 servings**

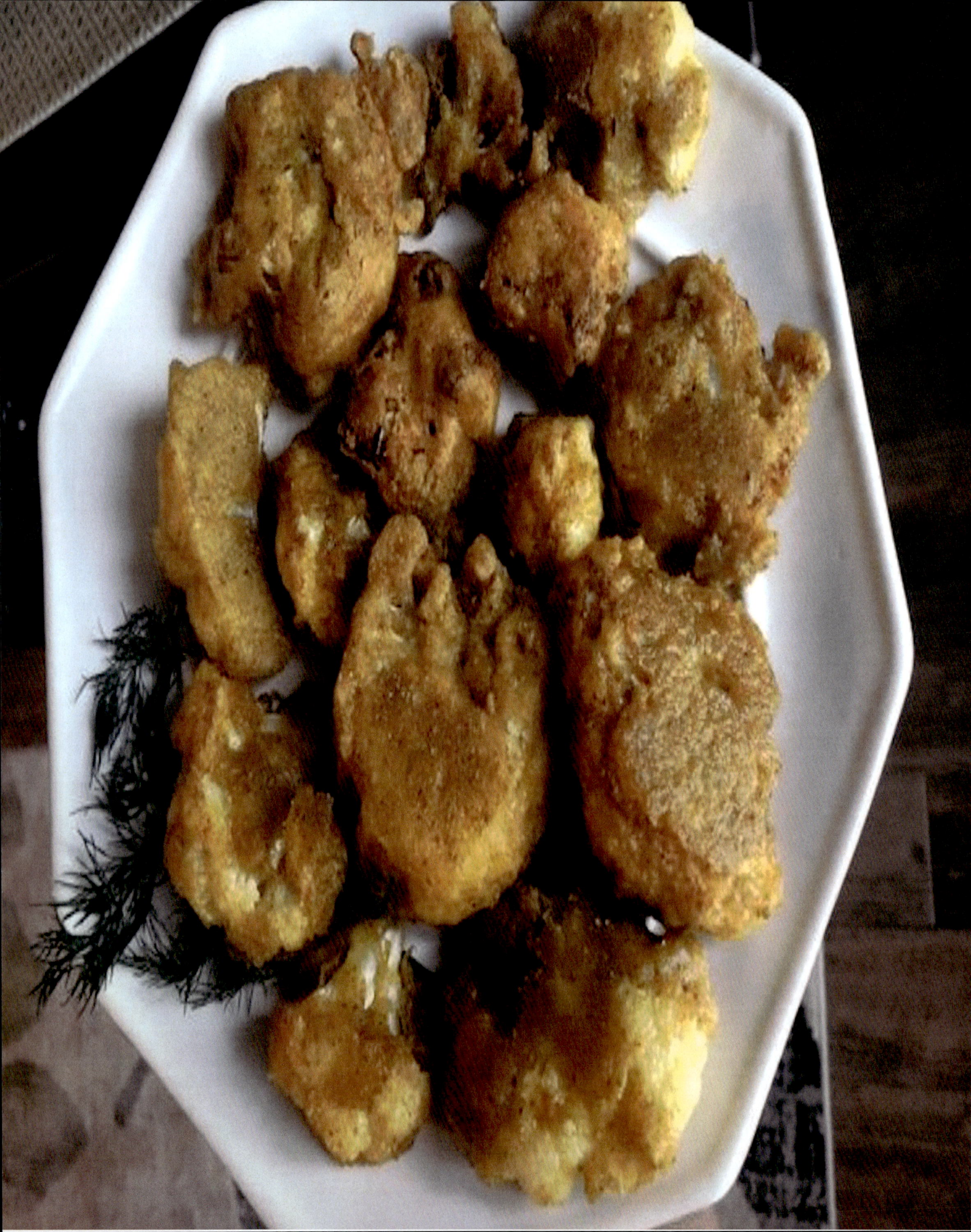

# Can't Believe It's Not Chicken Nuggets

**Ingredients:**

Batter mix (Pg39)

1 medium cauliflower (florets)

1 1/2 grapeseed oil

**Directions:**

In a skillet add the grapeseed oil over medium heat.

Next cut the cauliflower into florets. (**Cook's Tip:** Clean all veggies before eating them.)

In a medium-sized bowl, mix all the batter ingredients together until combined (pancake consistency).

Add the cauliflower florets to batter until fully coated with batter.

Next add cauliflower florets to skillet and cook 4-6 minutes until golden on each side. Transfer cook cauliflower florets onto a paper towel and let rest.

Delicious serve with your favorite sauce.

**Preparation time:20 minutes**
**Total time:35 minutes**
**Makes:3 servings**

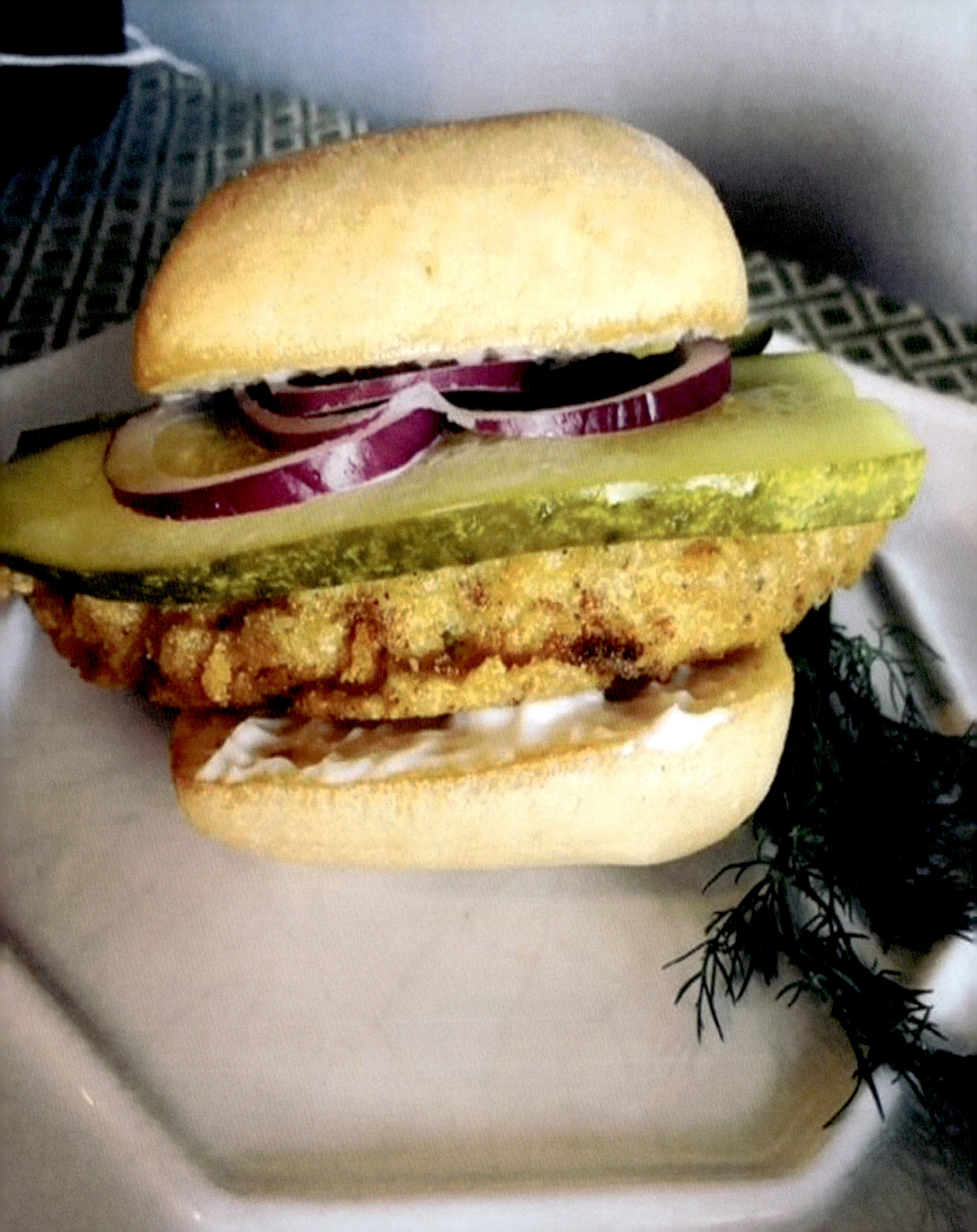

# Can't Believe It's Not A Chicken Sandwich

**Ingredients:**

1 medium cauliflower (steak cut)

1 vegan buns (O'Doughs) or your choice

2 slices dill pickles

1/2 cup red onions (sliced)

2 tsp vegan mayo (Just Mayo) or your choice

1 1/2 cup grapeseed oil

1/2 cup almond milk

1/2 tbsp vegan butter (Earth Balance) or your choice

**Batter Mix:**

10oz bag bread mix (New Orleans Seasonal Fish Fry) or your choice

1/2 cup corn meal

1/2 tsp garlic powder

1/2 tsp smoked paprika

1/2 ground chia seeds

1/2 tbsp starch

1/2 tsp Himalayan salt

1/2 tsp black pepper

1/2 cup almond milk (add more if it's too thick. Make it pancake consistency).

**Directions:**

In a skillet add the grapeseed oil over medium heat.

Next cut the cauliflower into steak slices. (**Cook's Tip:** Clean all vegetables before eating them.)

In a medium bowl, mix all the batter ingredients together until combined (pancake consistency). Add the cauliflower steak to batter until fully coated with batter. Next add cauliflower to skillet and cook 5-8 minutes on each side. Transfer cook cauliflower onto a paper towel and let rest.

Meanwhile, in a separate small skillet over medium heat. Cut the vegan buns in half and add butter on each side. Place buns in the skillet and cook for about 2-4 minutes on each side, then remove from skillet.

Transfer buns onto a plate. Add the mayo on each side of the bun. Place one cooked cauliflower on the bun. Add 1-2 two slices pickles and sliced red onions on top of cooked cauliflower.
Enjoy your Can't Believe It's Not Chicken Sandwich!

**Preparation time:20 minutes**
**Total time:35 minutes**
**Makes:4 servings**

***Reach Deeper***

*Reach deeper, don't be afraid of finding what you've been looking for, for a long time.*

*Reach deeper, it won't bite you, it won't even steal the essence of your emotional soul.*

*Reach deeper, if you reach deeper than the scars that were left behind, they won't keep you blind from the queen that you are.*

*Reach deeper, step into your divine radiant self-coloring the earth with your greatness.*

*Reach deeper, exhale in beauty, strength and confidence.*

*Reach Deeper.*

***Poetically Vegan***

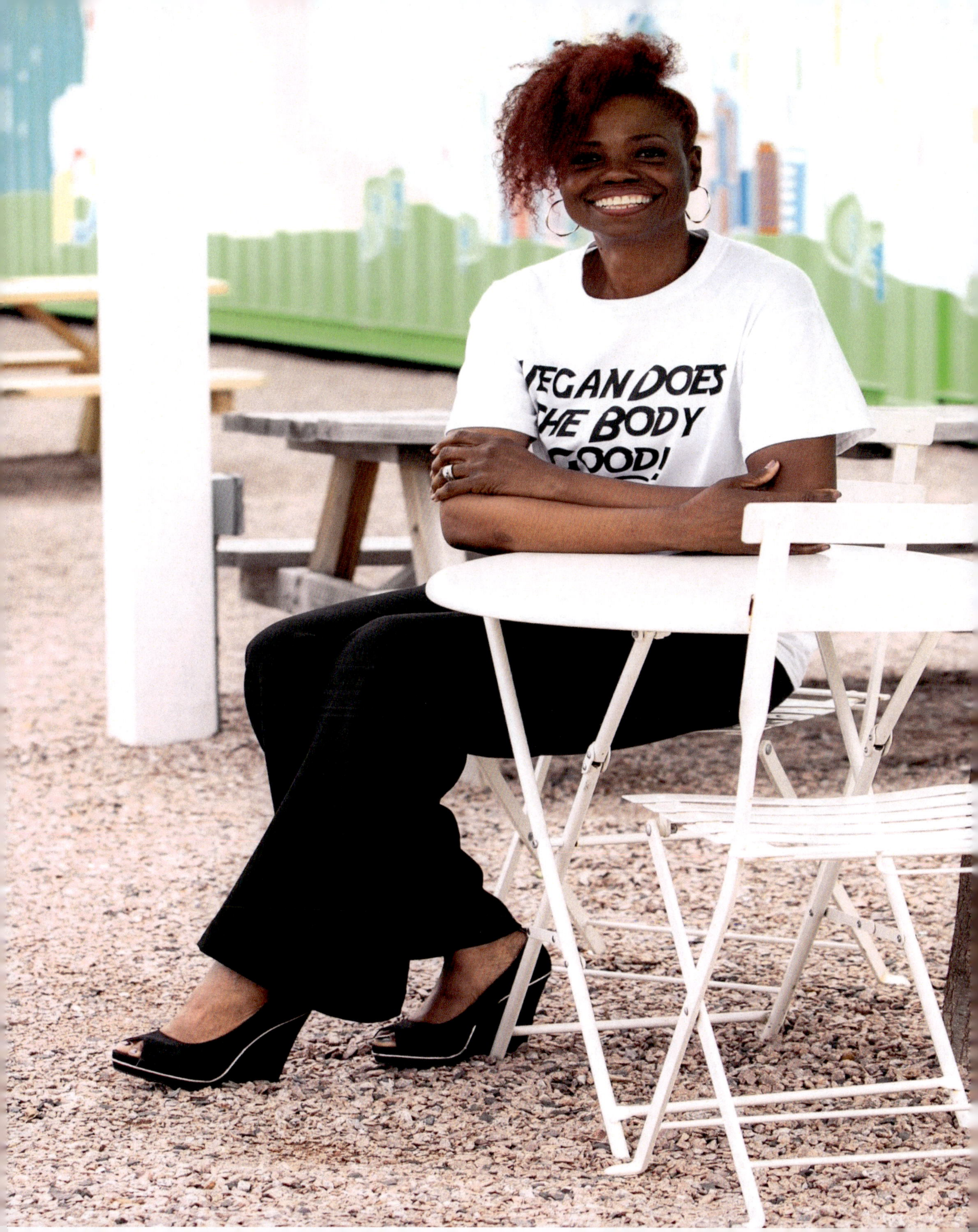
EGAN DOES
HE BODY
OOD!

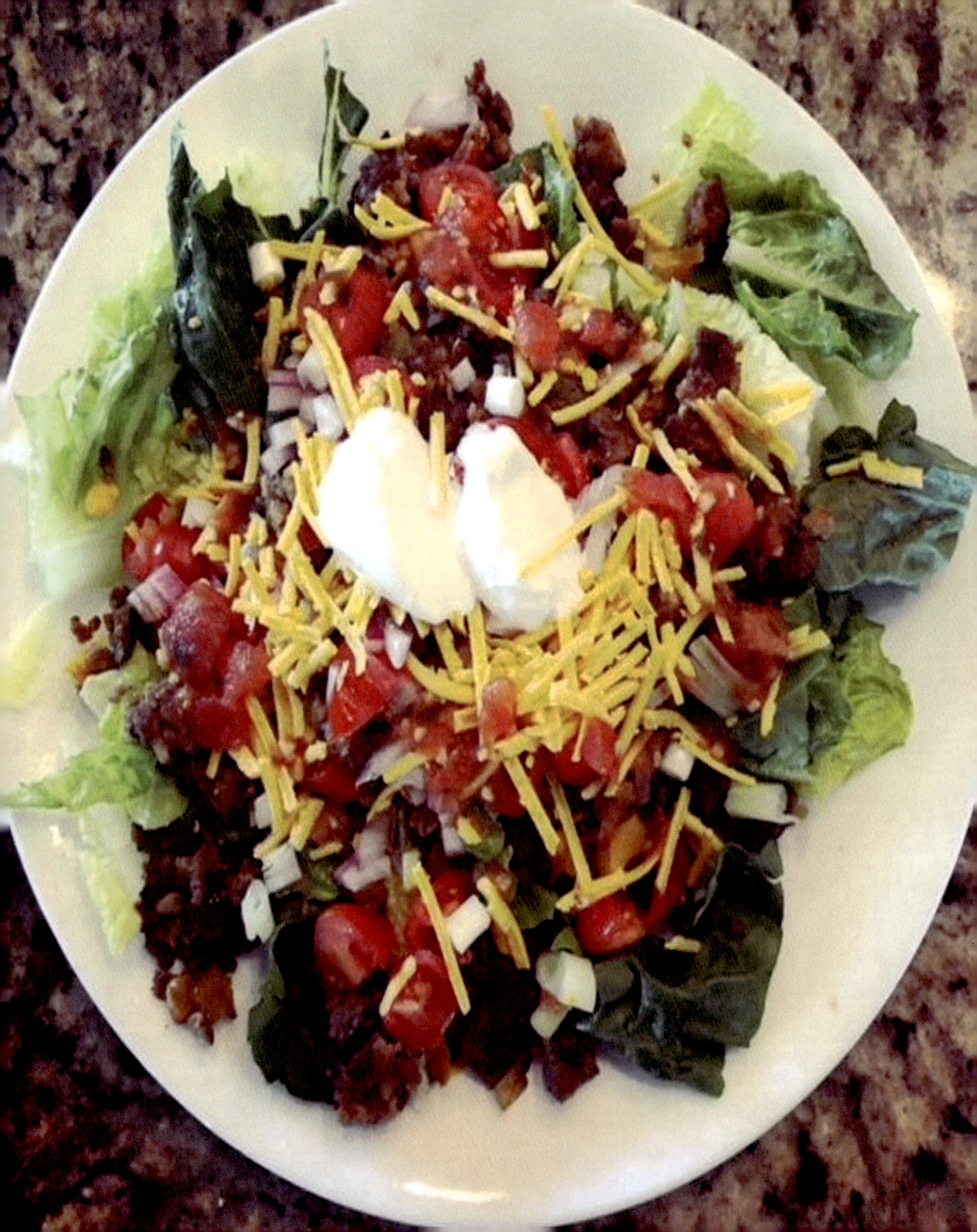

# Vegan Veggie Crumble Salad

**Ingredients:**

2 vegan veggie patty/crumble (Pg49)

1 1/2 cups chopped romaine lettuce

1 cup cherry tomatoes (sliced)

1/2 cup chopped red onions

1/2 cup vegan shredded cheese (Daiya) or your choice

2 tbsp vegan sour cream (Tofutti) or your choice

2 tbsp vegan salsa (Great Value) or your choice

**Directions:**

On a medium plate add the chopped romaine lettuce.

Add the vegan veggie crumble on top of the lettuce.

Add the sliced cherry tomatoes.

Add the chopped red onions.

Add the shredded cheese.

Add the salsa.

Add the sour cream.

Enjoy and don't forget to share!

**Preparation time:25**
**Total time:35 minutes**
**Makes:4 servings**

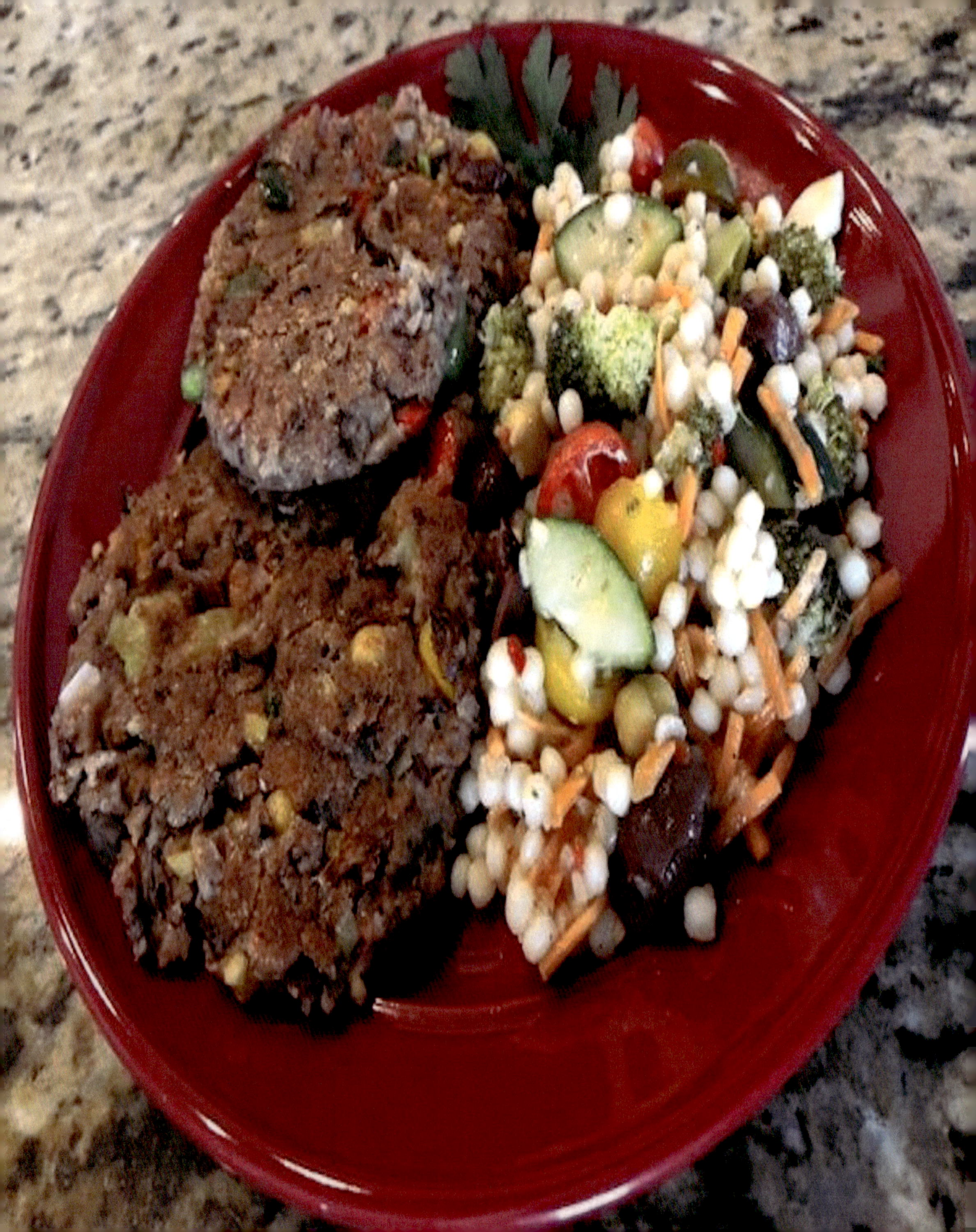

# Vegan Veggie Patty with Pearl Couscous Salad

**Ingredients:**

2 vegan veggie patty/crumble

1 cup pearl couscous

1 cup chopped cucumbers

1 cup slice melody cherry tomatoes

1/2 chopped red onions

1/2 cup kalamata olives (pitted and slice)

2 cups chopped broccoli

1 8-14 oz chickpeas (drained and rinsed)

1 1/2 cups shredded carrots

1 tsp Himalayan salt

1 tsp black pepper

**Dressing:**

4 Tbsp olive oil

1/2 tsp Himalayan salt

1/2 tsp black pepper

2 tsp lemon zest

2 garlic cloves, chopped, fresh grated garlic

Mix in a medium bowl until combined

**Directions:**

In a large mixing bowl add all the ingredients until mixed well.

Season to taste with Himalayan salt and black pepper.

Next place the two Vegan Veggie Patties on a plate with the Pearl Couscous Salad.

Garnish and Enjoy!

**Preparation time:20 minutes**
**Total time:35 minutes**
**Makes: 4 servings**

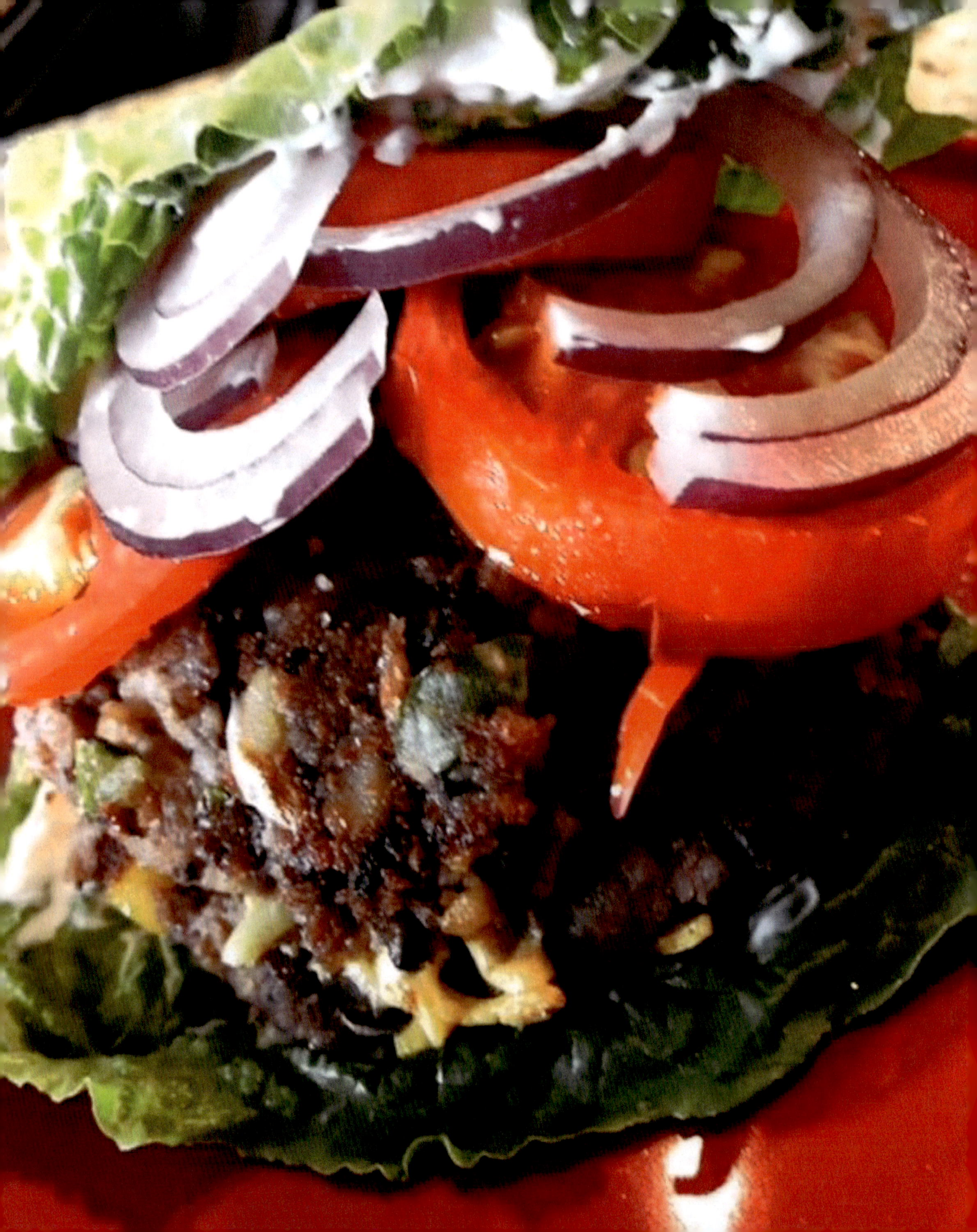

# Vegan Veggie Bunless Burger

**Ingredients:**

2 veggie patty/crumble (Pg49)

2 stacks of romaine lettuce

1oz red onions

2 slices of tomatoes

1 slice vegan cheese (Daiya) or your choice

2 tsp vegan mayo (Just Mayo) or your choice

**Directions:**

Form the mixer into 4-5 equal-size burgers. Let chill in the refrigerator for 30 minutes.

Add some of the mayo on the lettuce.

Add one patty on top of the lettuce.

Add one slice of vegan cheese on top of the patty.

Add the other patty on top of the vegan cheese.

Add the tomatoes on top of the veggie patty.

Add the sliced red onions on top of the tomatoes.

Add the rest of the vegan mayo on the lettuce and place the lettuce on top of the red onions.

Enjoy!

**Preparation time: 20 minutes**
**Total time: 35 minutes**
**Makes:4 servings**

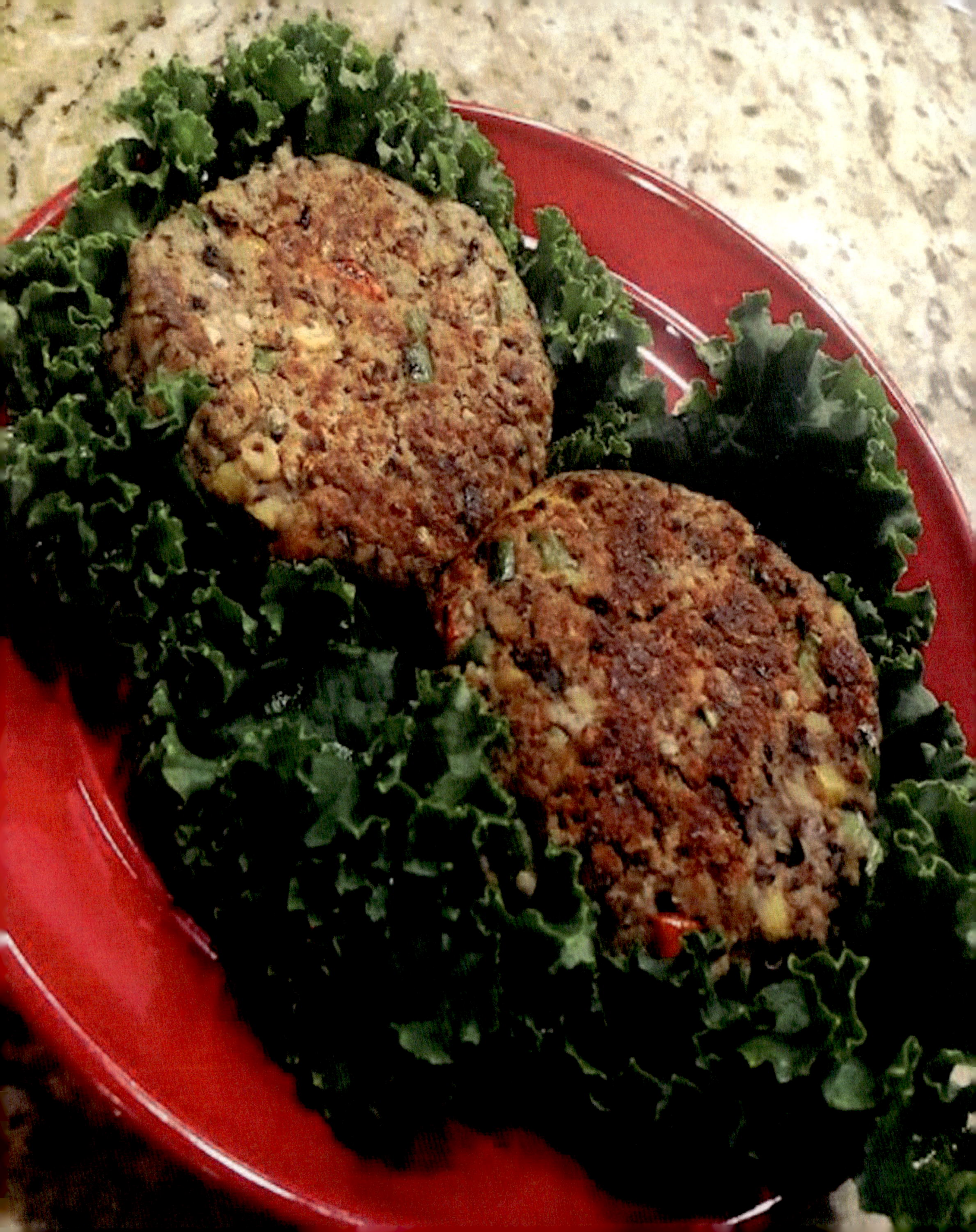

# Veggie Patty/Crumble

**Ingredients:**

1 10-14 oz can chickpea/garbanzo beans

1 10-14 oz can (BPA free) mixed beans

1 cup chopped red pepper

1 cup chopped yellow pepper

1 cup chopped green pepper

1 cup chopped orange pepper

1/2 red onions

1/2 green onions

1 cup chopped portobello mushrooms

1 1/2 cup spelt flour

1 1/2 cup breadcrumbs (Panko) or your choice

2 tbsp nutritional yeast (optional)

1 tsp Himalayan salt

1 tsp black pepper

1 tsp O bay seasoning

1 tsp smoked paprika

1 tsp liquid smoke

1 tbsp avocado oil

**Directions:**

In a large mixing bowl add the chickpeas and mixed beans. (**Cook's Tip:** Rinse and drain beans) Next mash the beans together with still a little texture to them. (**Cook's Tip:** When possible buy organic beans.

Add the red, yellow, green, orange bell peppers to the mixer. Add the red and green onions to the mixer.

Add the chopped portobello mushrooms, spelt flour and breadcrumbs and mix until combined.

Add all the spices to the mixture until combined.

Form the mixer into 4-5 equal-size burgers. Let chill in the refrigerator for 30 minutes.

Next form 4-6oz of the mixture into a patty. Let chill in the refrigerator for 30 minutes.

Place the patty in the skillet with the avocado oil and cook for about 5 mins on each side until golden.

Remove from skillet and place on paper towel.

Serve warm or room temperature. Enjoy!

**Preparation time:20 minutes**
**Total time:35 minutes**
**Makes: 4 servings**

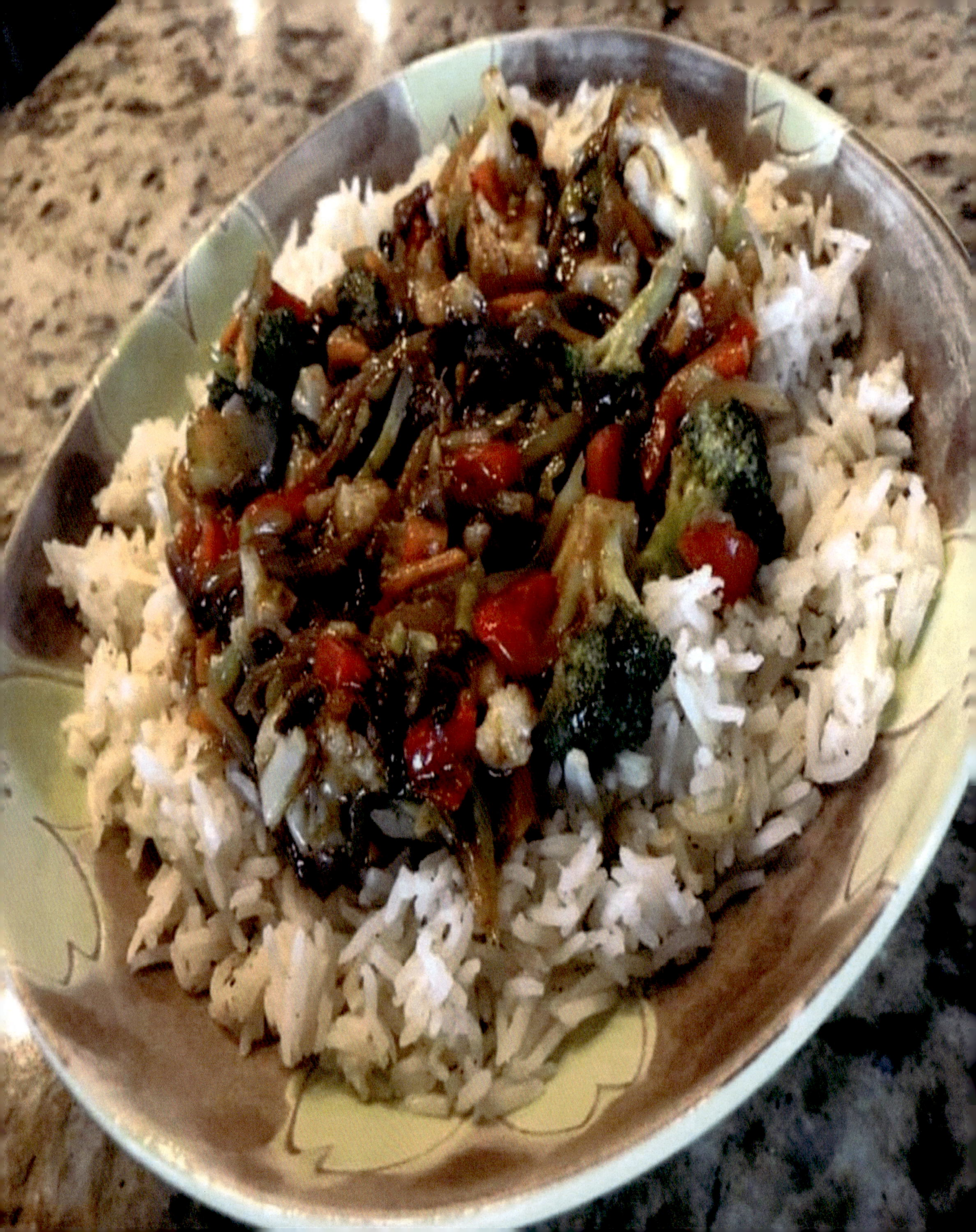

# Vegan Thai-Style Buddha Bowl/Plate

**Ingredients:**

1 cup basmati rice (cook according to directions)

1/2 green bell pepper (chopped)

1/2 red bell pepper (chopped)

1 cup broccoli (chopped)

1 cup zucchini (chopped)

1/2 cup broccoli and carrot slaw

1/2 red onions (chopped)

1/2 cup vegan Thai sauce (or make it homemade)

Add pinch of Himalayan salt & black pepper for more flavor (optional)

1 tbsp grapeseed oil or 1/2 cup vegan vegetable broth

**Directions:**

In a medium skillet add the grapeseed oil. Add the onions, broccoli and carrot slaw, broccoli, green bell pepper, red bell pepper, zucchini, Himalayan salt and black pepper (optional). Stir until combine. Don't overcook the mixture, make with a little crush to taste.

Add 1/2 cup Thai sauce to the skillet. Stir the mixture until combine.

In a medium bowl/plate add the basmati rice. Add the mixture on top of the rice.

Enjoy!

**Preparation time:20 minutes**
**Total time:30 minutes**
**Makes:2 servings**

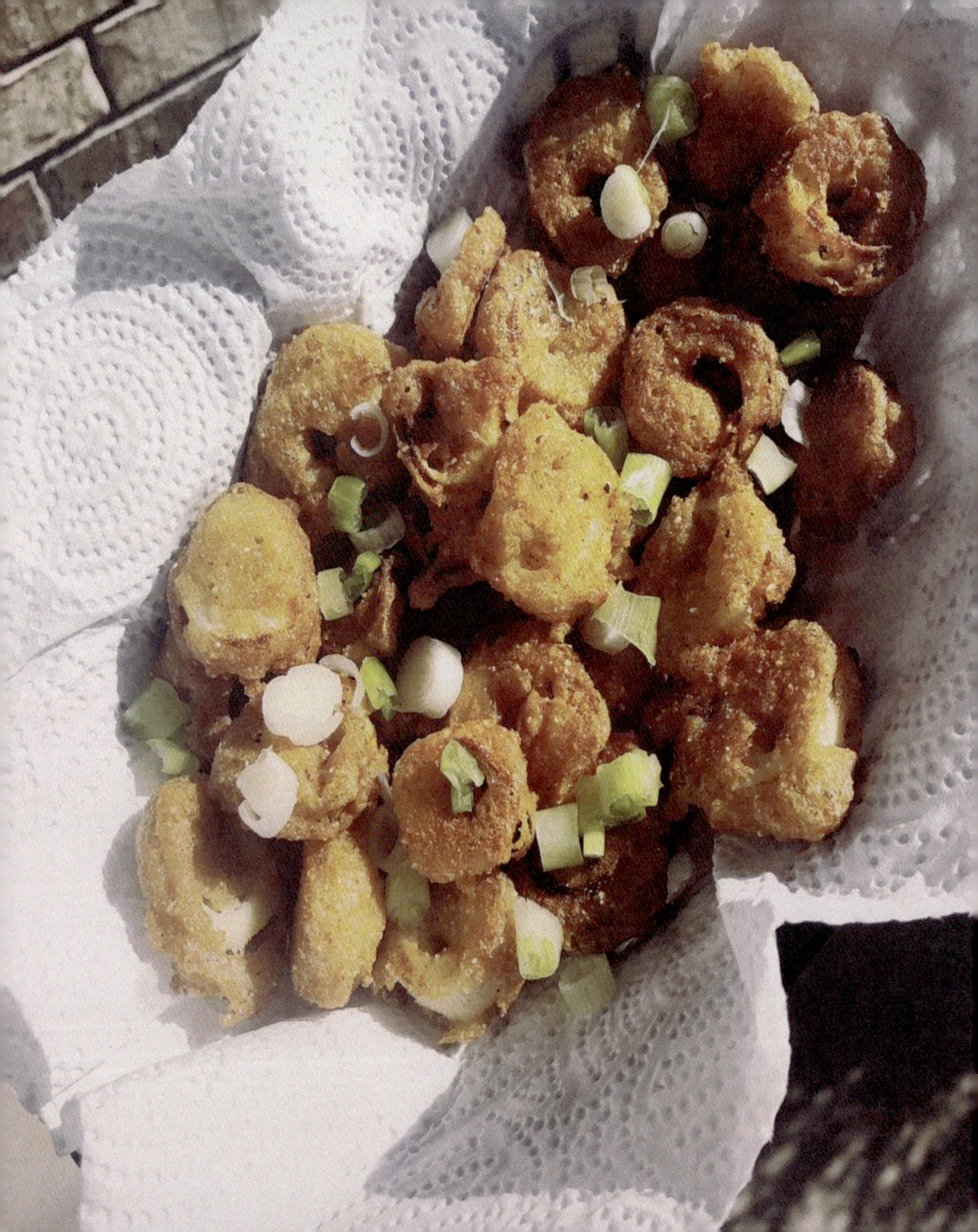

# Spicy Vegan Calamari

**Ingredients:**

Use Batter on Pg.39

1 14oz can hearts of palm (drained, sliced, and middle removed)

1/2 tsp Himalayan salt

1/2 tsp black pepper

1 tsp old bay seasonings

1/2 tsp garlic powder

1/2 tsp onion powder

1 1/2 cup grapeseed oil

(**Cook Tip**: Do not throw away the juice from the hearts of palm. It can be used to add to batter mixture if needed).

**Directions:**

In a medium saucepan add the grapeseed oil on medium heat.

In a medium bowl, add the sliced hearts of palm. Add the Himalayan salt, black pepper, old bay seasonings, garlic powder, onion powder. Mix the ingredients well.

In a medium bowl prepare the batter mixture. Add the hearts of palm to the mixture only a few at a time.

Make sure to coat the hearts of palm well.

Place about 4-5 pieces of the sliced hearts of palm in the oil. Fry the hearts of palm until golden brown, about 3-5 minutes on each side. Remove fried hearts of palm with a slotted spoon and place on a paper towel.

Garnish with fresh green onions. Enjoy!

**Preparation time:20 minutes**
**Total time:30 minutes**
**Makes:2 servings**

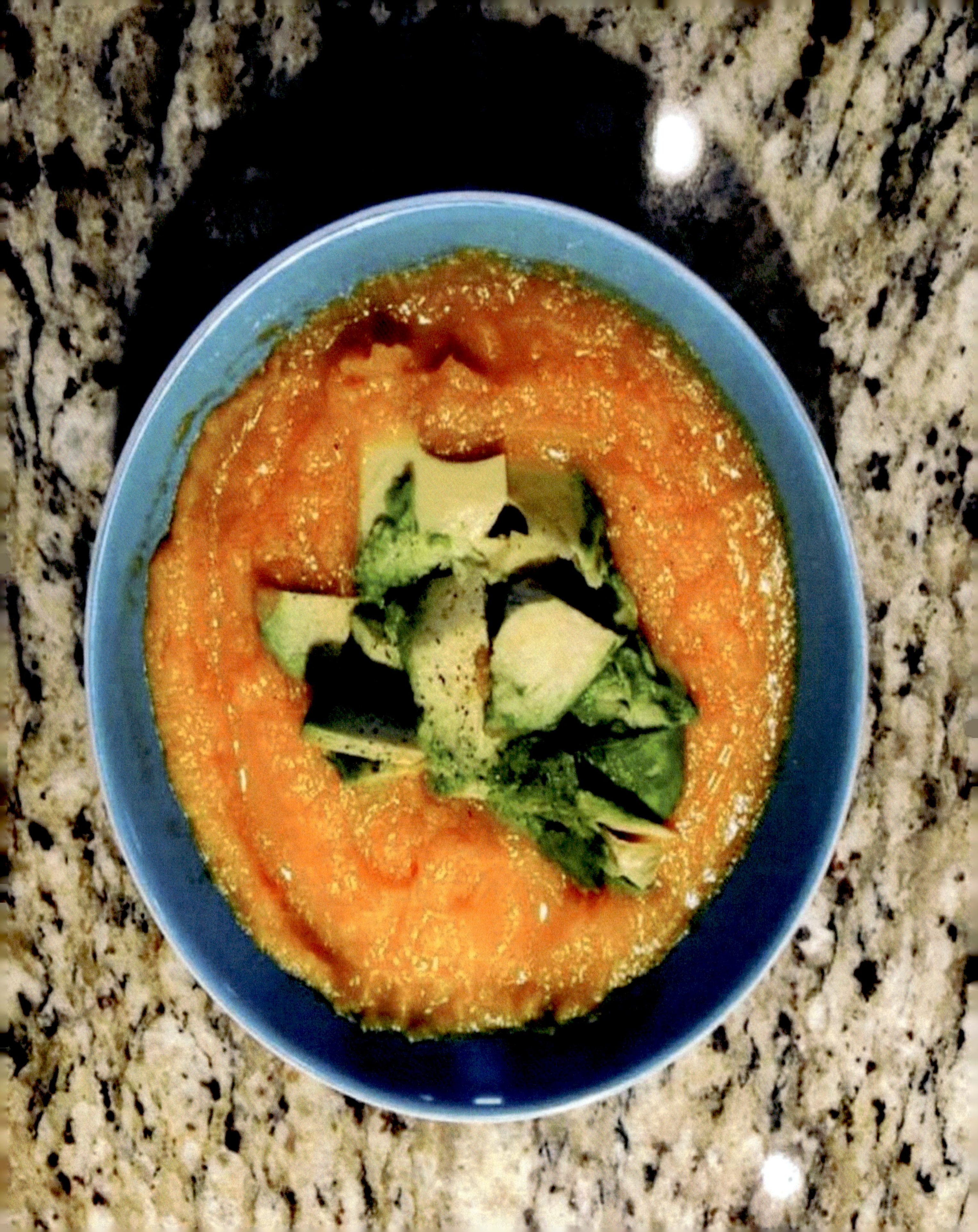

# Roasted Butternut Squash Soup

**Ingredients:**

1 medium to large butternut squash

1 tbsp grapeseed oil

1/2 tsp Himalayan salt

1/2 tsp black pepper

1/2 cup almond milk (add more if needed)

1/3 cup vegetable broth

2 tbsp vegan sour cream (Tofutti milk free) or your choice

**to garnish:**

optional, plain vegan yogurt (Kite Hill plain) or your choice

**Directions:**

Preheat the oven to 350°F.

Scrub the butternut squash and place on a baking sheet. Prick the butternut; squash all over with a fork and rub the oil into the skin.

Cook in the preheated oven for 45-60 minutes, or until soft.

Using a sharp knife, cut the butternut squash in half lengthwise and scoop out the seeds.

Next scoop out the flesh into a food processor or blender. Add Himalayan salt, black pepper, almond milk, vegetable broth, and vegan sour cream. Process until smooth.

Transfer the soup to a medium serving bowl, garnish with swirls of vegan yogurt and pinch of Himalayan salt and black pepper.

**Serve at once and enjoy!**

**Preparation time:20 minutes**
**Total time:40 minutes**
**Makes:4 servings**

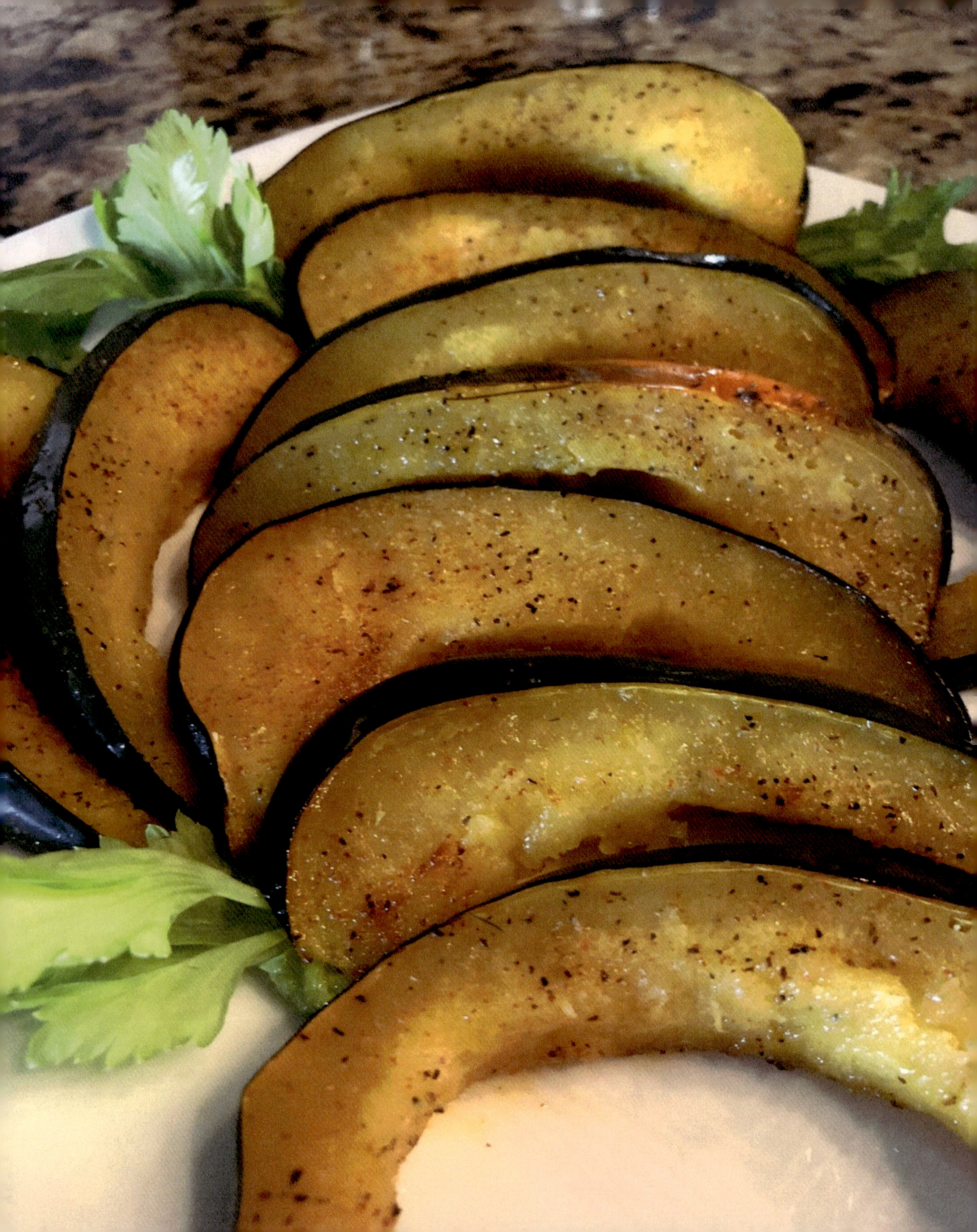

# Roasted Acorn Squash Wedges

**Ingredients:**

2 small to medium acorn squash

1 1/2 tbsp grapeseed oil

1/2 tsp Himalayan salt

1/2 tsp black pepper

1/2 garlic powder

1/2 onion powder

1/2 tsp smoked paprika powder

**Directions:**

Preheat the oven to 350°F. Scrub the acorn squash. Using a sharp knife, cut the acorn into half and scoop out the seeds. Using a sharp knife cut the squash into wedges and place on a baking sheet.

Next sprinkle the oil, Himalayan salt, black pepper, garlic powder, onion powder, paprika powder on the acorn wedges both sides.

Bake in the preheated oven for about 35-45 minutes or until soft, then transfer to a serving platter and enjoy.

(**Cook Tip:** Leftovers can be eaten for a snack room temp or warm.)

**Preparation time:20 minutes**
**Total time:35 minutes**
**Makes:3 servings**

***Dreams***

*Who said my dreams were only on paper*

*Just because your dreams sat on paper and the ink faded away*

*Now you can't even see what was meant to be*

*Your dreams are hanging in the memory of an iCloud, no access to that file*

*Dreams are to be filled and not left in the field of no hope*

*Don't let the world water down your dreams thinking their unreachable*

*Even Martin Luther King had a dream*

*He dreamed that one day the rough places will be made plain and the crooked places will be made straight*

*So, I need for you to create*

*We all have had dreams that tried to escape*

*But with valor, endurance, perseverance there's a way*

*So, I'm here to tell you*

*Dreams do come true, because I See You*

***Poetically Vegan***

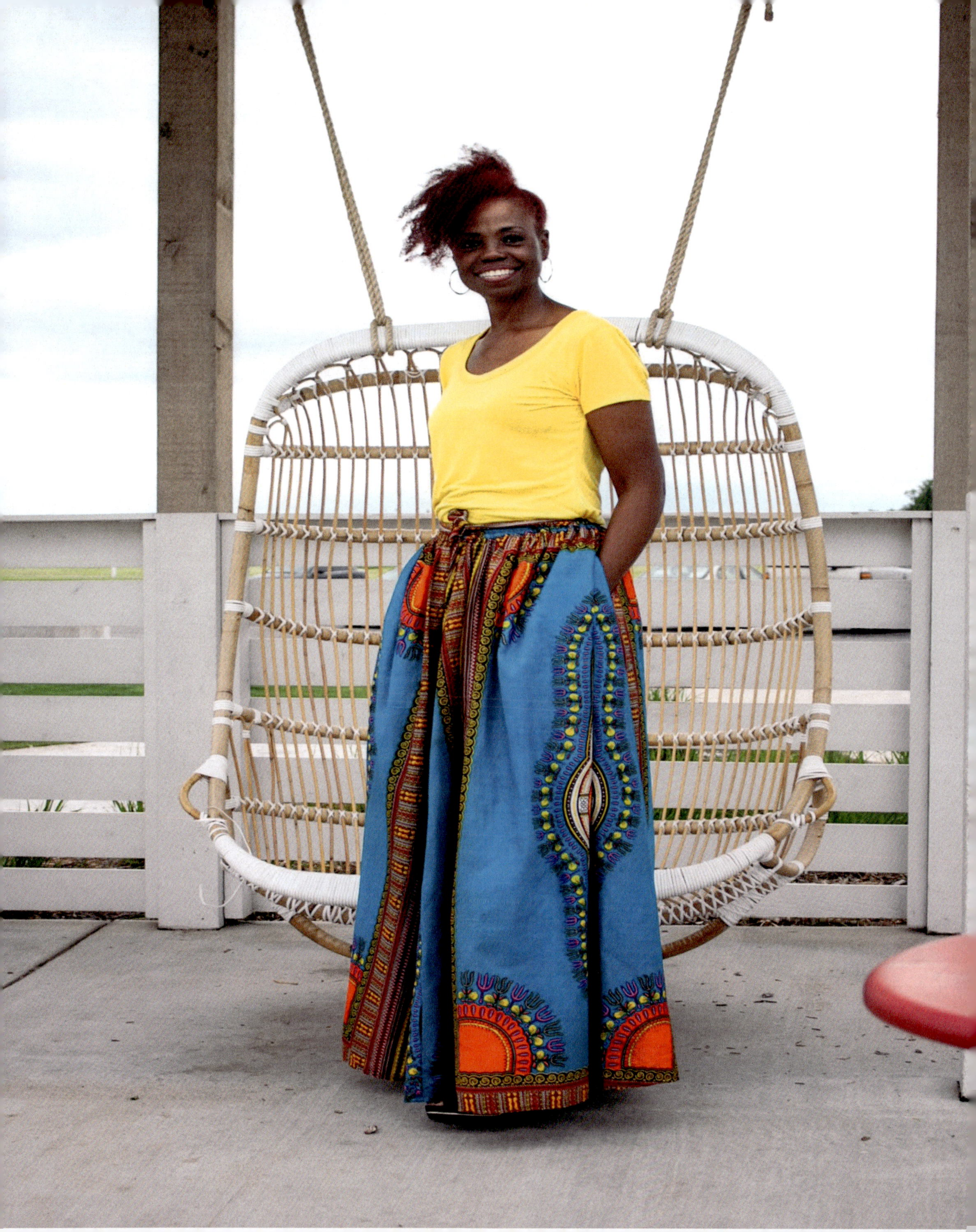

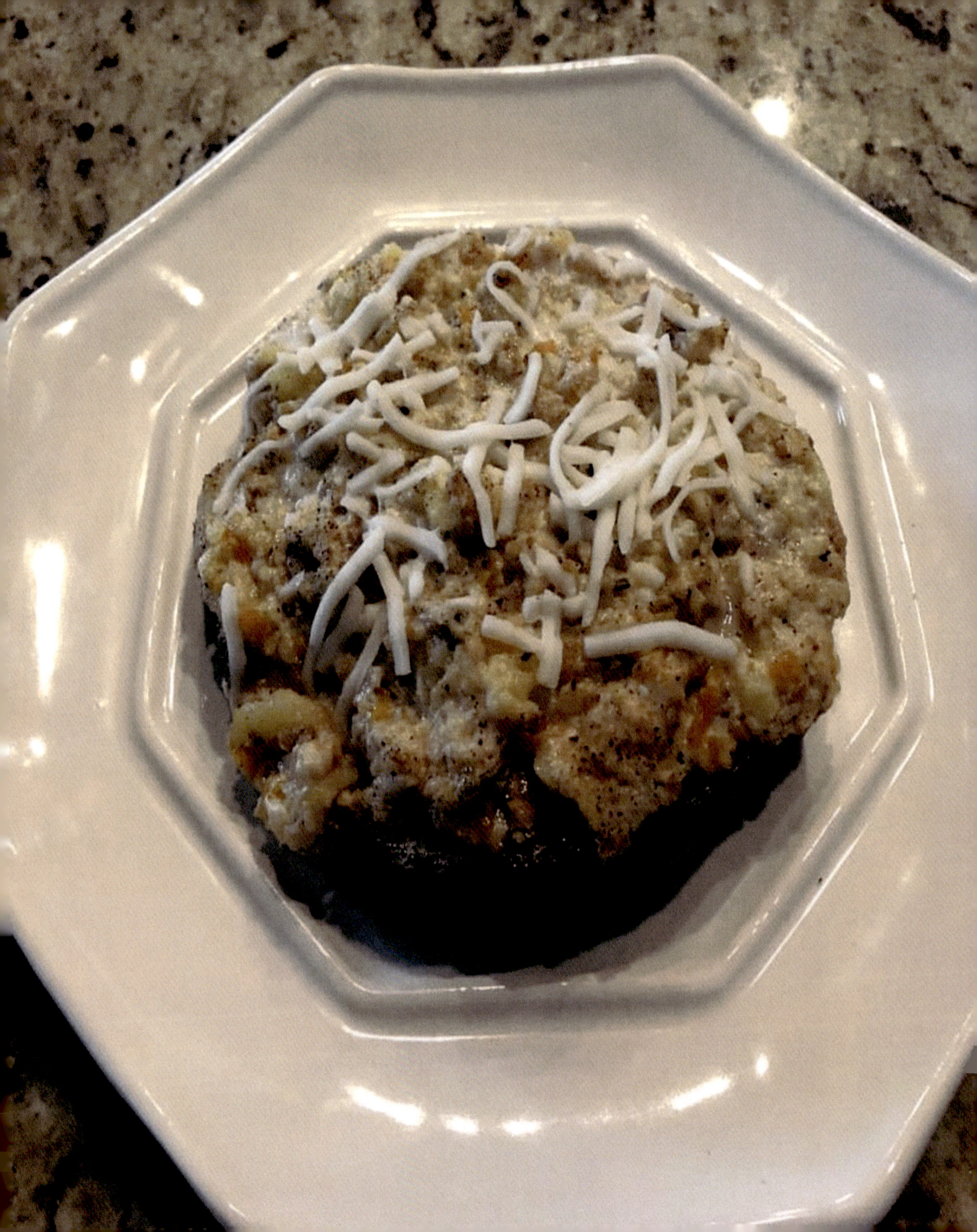

# Stuffed Portobello Mushrooms

**Ingredients:**

2 medium organic portobello mushrooms (clean mushrooms and remove stalks)

Vegan Double Baked Yukon Potatoes (leftover mixture)

1 tbsp grape seed oil (vegan butter optional)

1 tsp Himalayan salt

1 black pepper

**Directions:**

Pre-heat the oven to 325°F.

Place the mushrooms on a baking sheet. Spread the grape seed oil on the mushroom.

Sprinkle Himalayan salt, pepper, and spoon the mixture into the mushroom.

Bake for 15-20 minutes.

Transfer the baked mushroom on to serving plates and serve at once.

**Preparation time:15 minutes**
**Total time:35 minutes**
**Makes:4 servings**

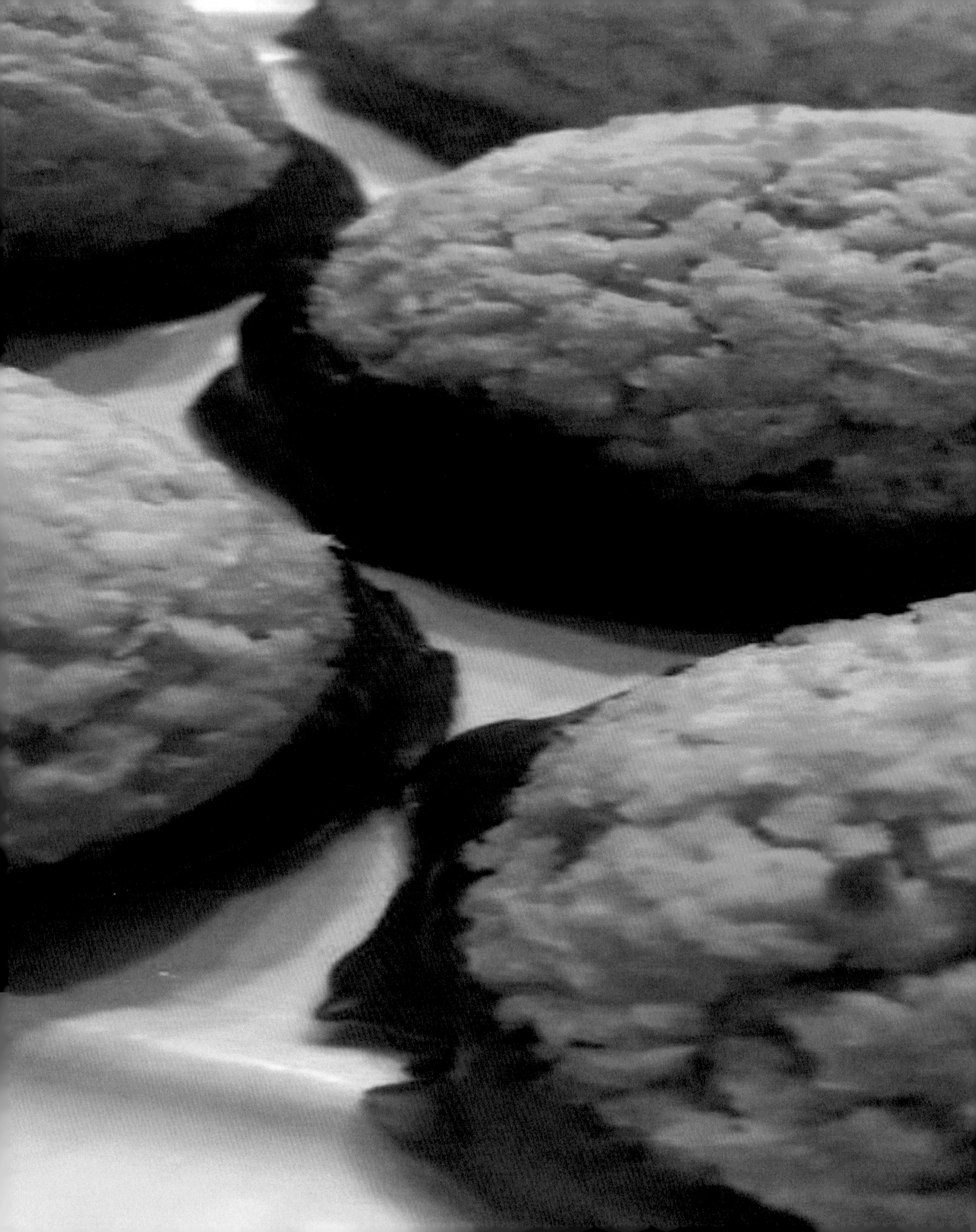

# *DESSERTS*

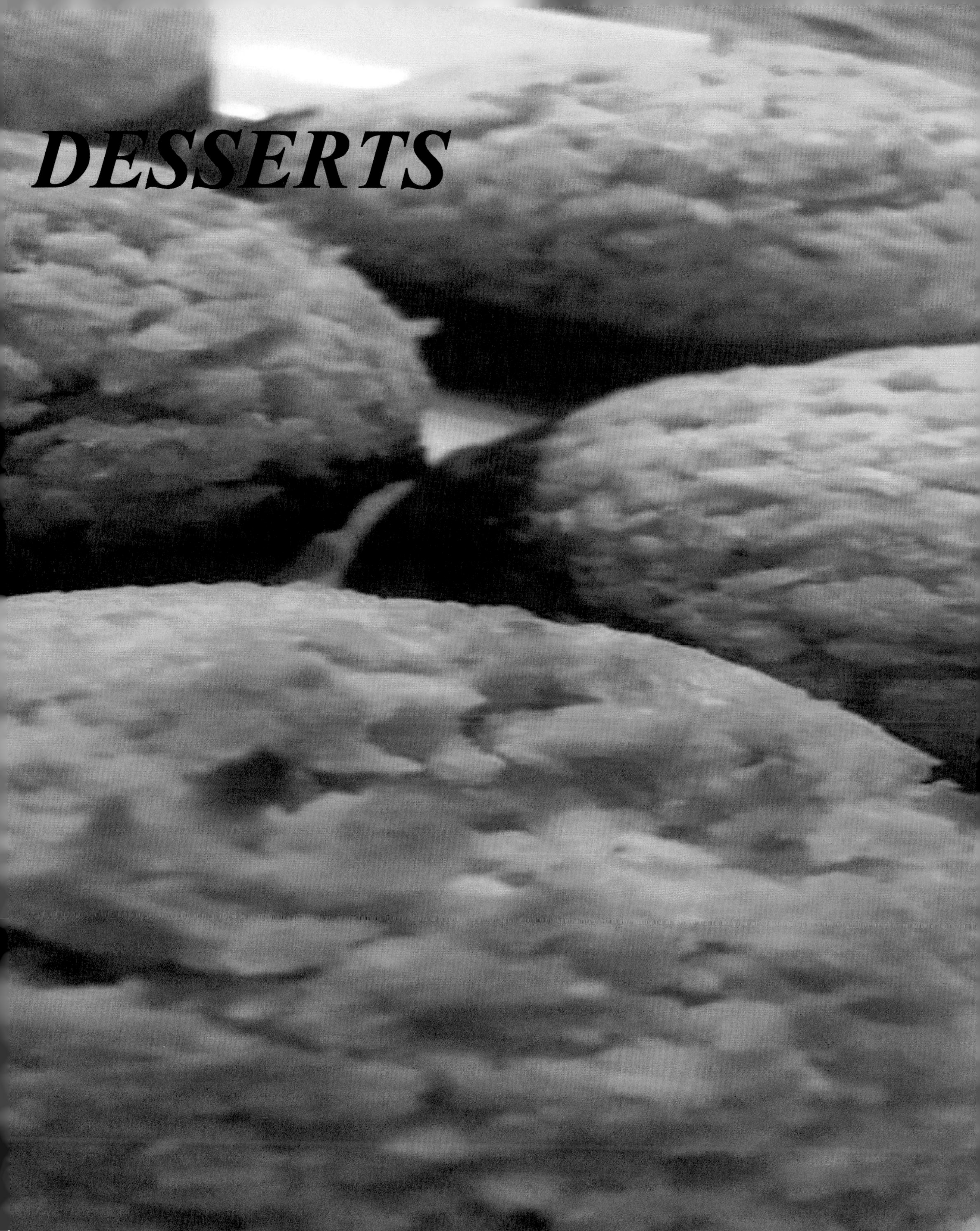

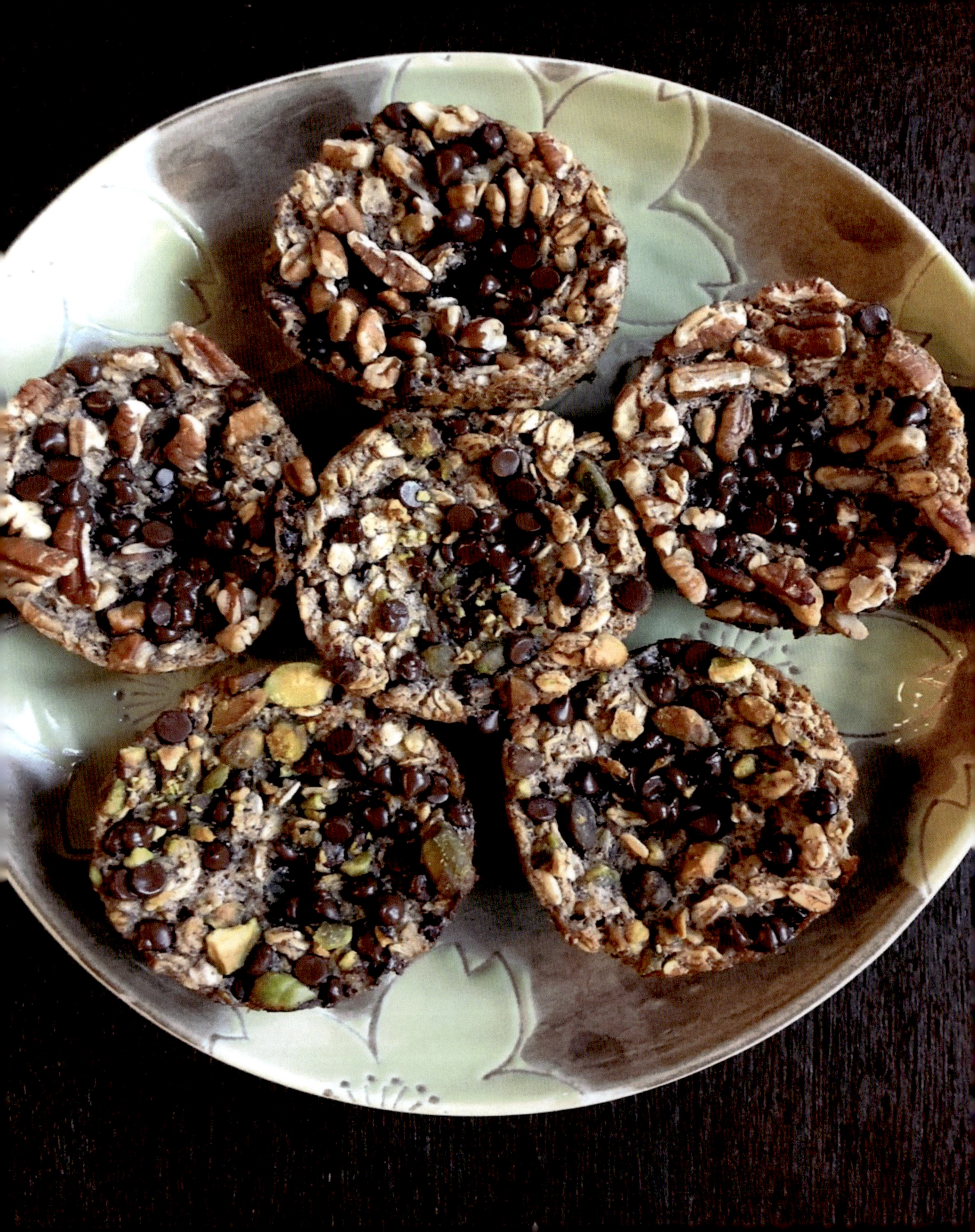

# Chocolate Chip Banana Nut Muffins

**Ingredients:**

2 1/2 cups rolled oats (Organic and no GMO)

2 tsp baking powder

1 tsp cinnamon

2 tbsp. date or coconut sugar date sugar

1/4 tsp ground nutmeg

1/2 tsp kosher or Himalayan salt

1/2 tsp vanilla extract

2 tbsp ground/meal flax seed or ground chia seeds

2 flax eggs (6 tbsp water and 2 tbsp of ground/meal flax seeds)

1 cup chopped pecans

1 cup masked ripped bananas (2-3 bananas)

2 tbsp mini chocolate chip (vegan)

**Directions:**

1. In a medium bowl combine roll oats, baking powder, coconut sugar or date sugar, ground nutmeg, cinnamon, ground flax seed/chia, kosher/Himalayan salt, mix well.

2. Add masked ripped bananas, chopped pecans,

chocolate chips, vanilla extract, flax eggs.

3. Combine all the ingredients.

4. Preheat oven to 350°F and prepare your muffin cups with oil (coconut, grapeseed, avocado).

4. Add spoonful of ingredients to each muffin cups.

5. Bake 20-35 minutes.

Great snack on the go!

**Preparation time:20 minutes**
**Total time:35 minutes**
**Makes:8 servings**

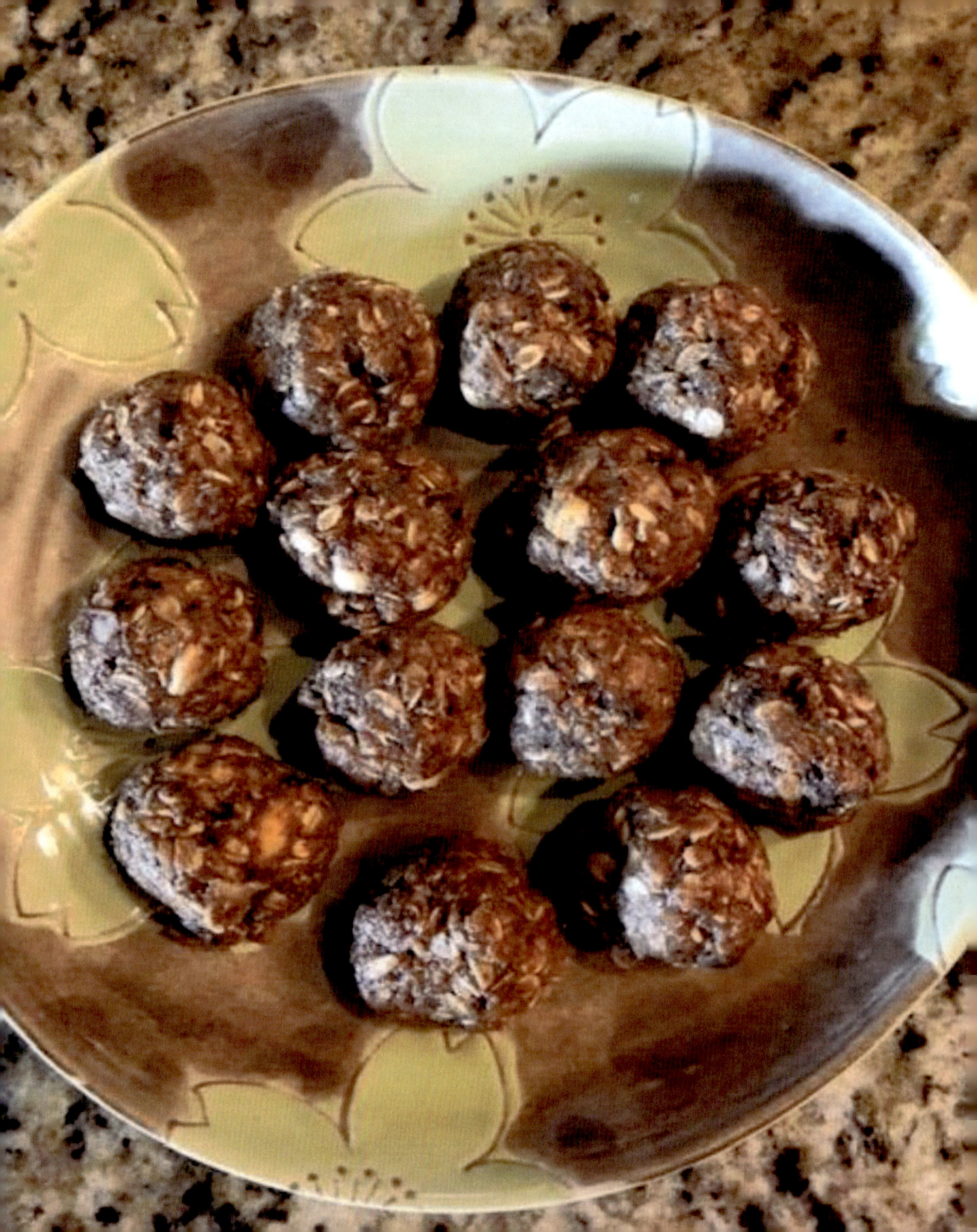

# Vegan Cashews Chocolate Chip Protein Balls

**Ingredients:**

2 cups organic roll oats

1/2 cup organic peanut butter

1 tsp cinnamon

1 tbsp maple syrup

1/2 cup chocolate chips

1/2 cup cashews (chopped)

**Directions:**

In a medium bowl add the roll oats, cinnamon, chocolate chip, peanut butter, maple syrup, and cashews. Mixed until combined.

Roll ingredients into small to medium balls.

Place into your favorite container.

Chill for 30 minutes.

Good, Easy, Simple to Make at Home! Enjoy!

**Preparation time:15 minutes**
**Total time:20 minutes**
**Makes:10 servings**

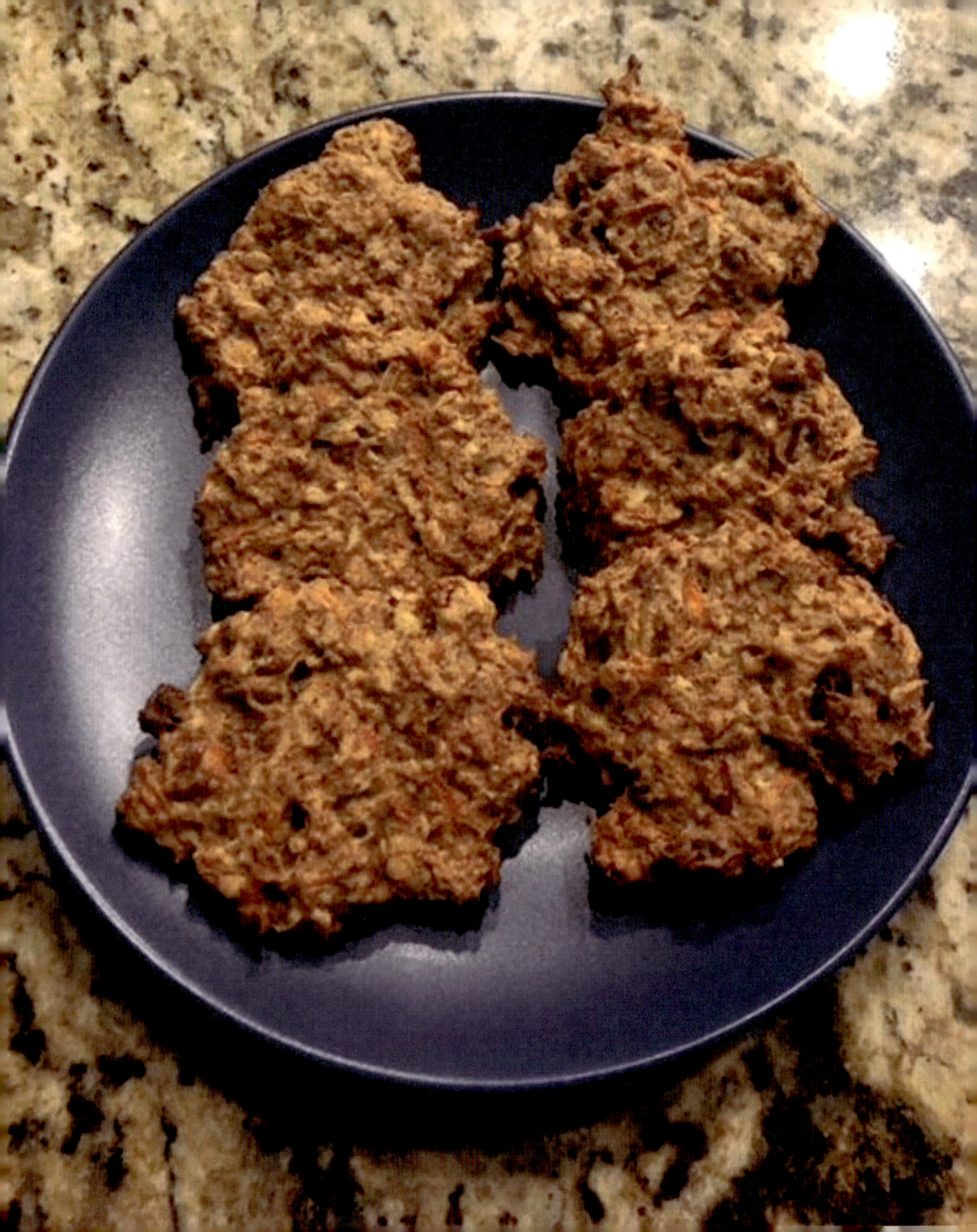

# Apple Carrot Cookies

**Ingredients:**

1 1/2 cup whole wheat flour

1 cup old fashioned oats

1/2 cup pecans

1 1/2 tsp baking power

1/2 tsp baking soda

1 tsp ground cinnamon

1/4 nutmeg

1/4 coconut oil

1/4 pinch Himalayan salt

3/4 cup grated carrot

3/4 cup grated apple

2 eggs (2 tbsp ground flax seeds and 6 tbsp of water)

1/3 cup maple syrup

2 tsp pure vanilla extract

**Directions:**

Heat your oven to 350°F.

Lightly spray cookie sheet with non-stick spray (coconut oil).

Add all dry ingredients in a large bowl mixed well.

Add the grated carrot and apple and fold to combine.

Add all wet ingredients in a medium bowl whisk together.

Add the wet ingredients to the dry ingredients, stir gently until just combine. Do not over mix.

Drop by rounded tablespoonfuls onto cookie sheet.

Bake for 10-15 minutes until desired doneness. Allow to cool fully.

**Preparation time:15 minutes**
**Total time:30 minutes**
**Makes:8 servings**

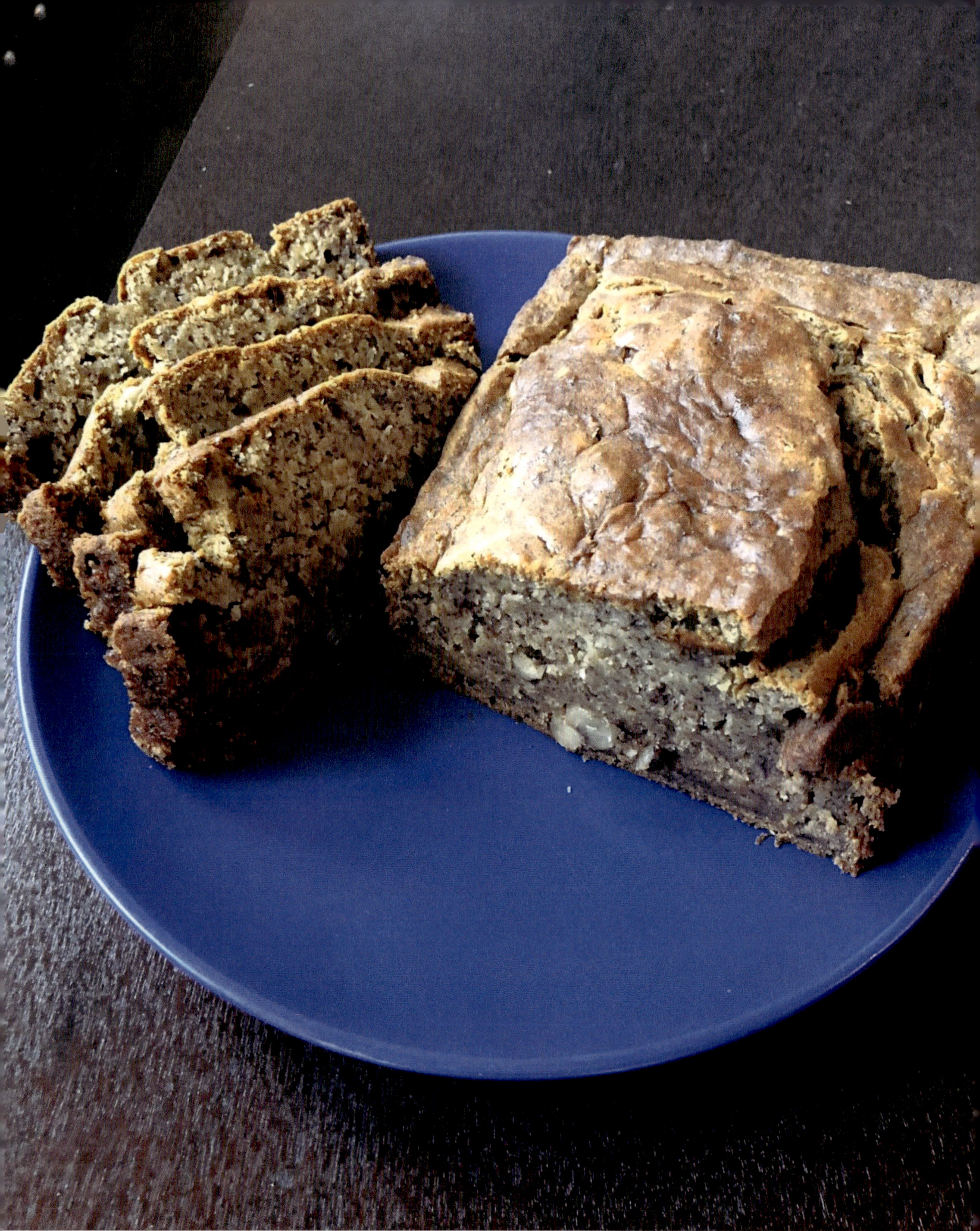

# Vegan Banana Walnut Bread

**Ingredients:**

1 1/4 cup wheat flour

1 tsp baking soda

pinch of Kosher salt

1 cup maple flakes or 3/4 cup maple syrup

1/2 cup melted vegan butter

1/4 cup almond milk (or any plant-based milk)

1 tbsp vanilla extract

2 flax eggs (2 tbs of ground flax/ chia seeds and 6 tbs of water)

3 large ripped bananas, mashed

1/2 cup slightly chopped walnuts

**Directions:**

Preheat oven to 350°

Spray 9"X5" Loaf pan with coconut spray.

In a large bowl mix together all dry ingredients.

In another large bowl mix together all wet ingredients including the walnuts and bananas.

Pour wet ingredients over dry and stir until combined.

Transfer the batter to prepared pan.

Bake about 1 hour or a toothpick comes out clean.

Add melted vegan butter on top (optional), Cool (or eat warm), Serve, & Enjoy!

**Preparation time:20 minutes**
**Total time:35 minutes**
**Makes:6 servings**

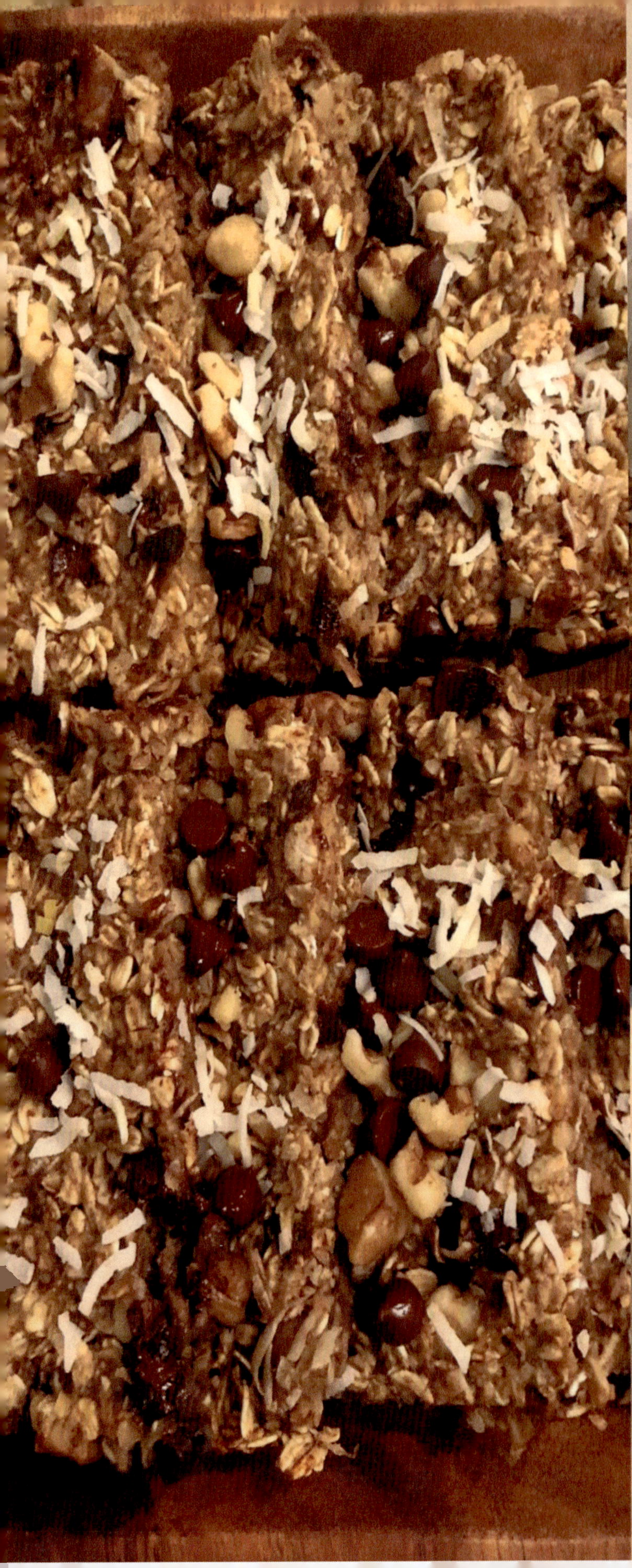

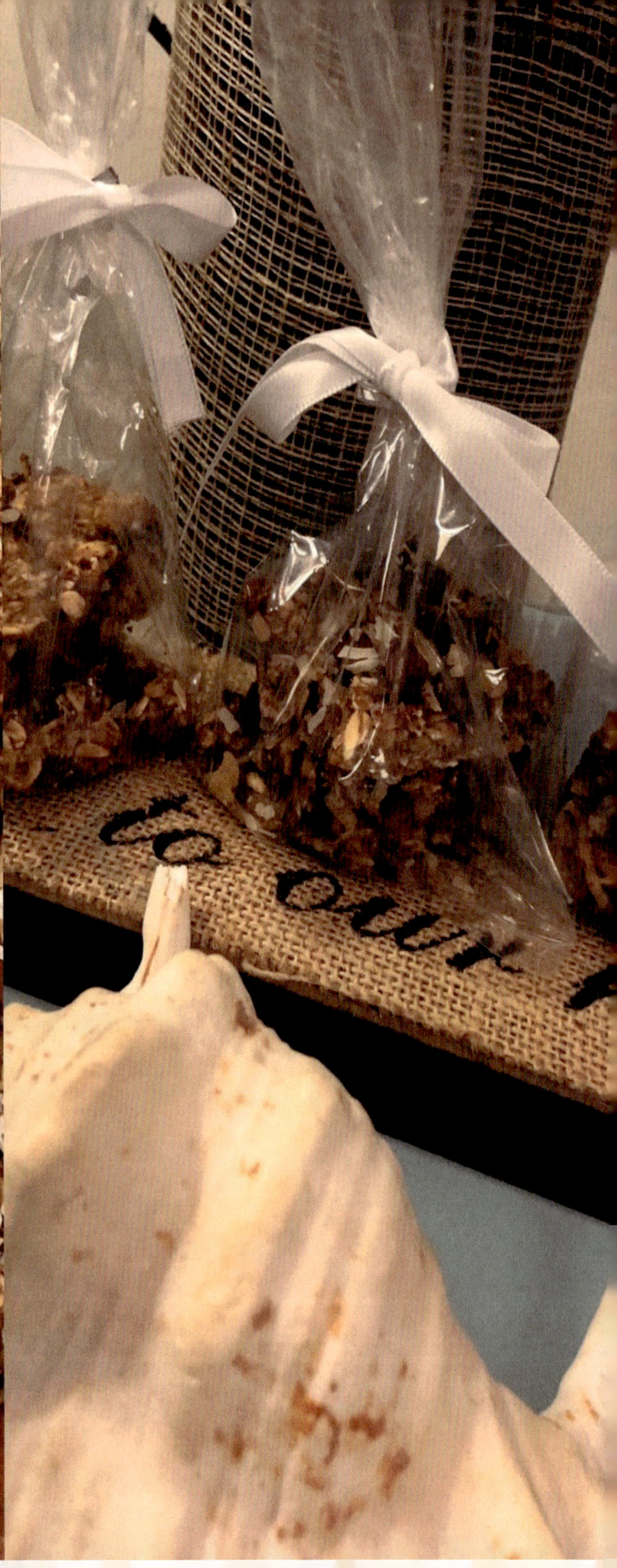

# Vegan Coconut Chocolate Chip Walnut Squares

**Ingredients:**

2 1/2 cups rolled oats (Organic and no GMO)

2 tsp baking powder

1 tsp cinnamon

2 tbsp date or coconut sugar date sugar

2 tbsp monk fruit sweetener

1/4 tsp ground nutmeg

1/2 tsp kosher or Himalayan salt

1/2 tsp vanilla extract

2 flax eggs (6 tbsp water and 2 tbsp. of ground/meal flax seeds)

1 cup walnut (chopped)

1 cup shredded coconut

1 cup masked ripped bananas (2-3 bananas)

1 cup mini chocolate chip (vegan)

**Directions:**

In a medium bowl combine roll oats, baking powder, coconut sugar or date sugar, monk fruit sweetener, ground nutmeg, cinnamon, kosher/Himalayan salt, mix well.

Add masked ripped bananas, walnuts, shredded coconut, chocolate chips, vanilla extract, flax eggs.

Combine all the ingredients.

Preheat oven to 350 f and prepare medium sheet pan with oil or non-stick spray (coconut, grapeseed,avocado).

Add ingredients to a medium sheet pan and spread evenly.

Bake 20-35 minutes, cool for 10-15 minutes and cut in small to medium squares.

Garnish with shredded coconut, chocolate chips, and walnuts (optional)

Enjoy!

**Preparation time:15 minutes**
**Total time:30 minutes**
**Makes:8 servings**

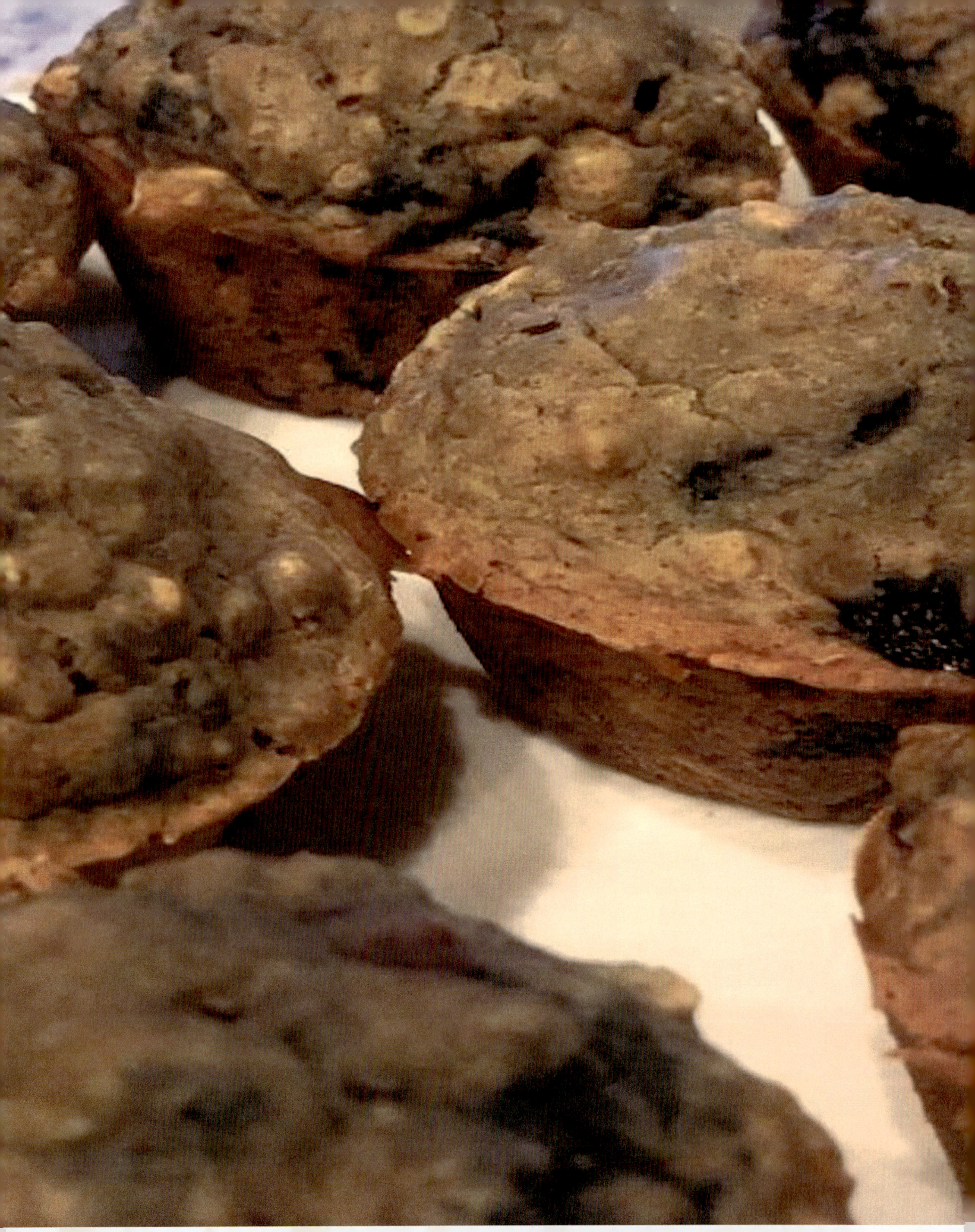

# Vegan Blueberry Coconut Yogurt Muffins

**Ingredients:**

1 cup all-purpose flour (organic-unbleached)

1 cup old fashioned oats

1/2 tsp baking soda

1 1/2 tsp baking powder

1 tsp cinnamon

2 tsp vanilla extract

2 tbsp coconut oil

1/4 tsp kosher salt

1/2 cup coconut sugar

1 flax egg

1 cup blueberry yogurt

1/2 cup coconut milk

1 1/2 cup fresh or frozen blueberries

Icing: (optional)

8 tbsp vegan butter (room temperature)

1 1/2 cup Vegan powdered sugar

1/2 vanilla extract

Place all ingredients in a mixing bowl blend until soften and fluffy using a hand mixer.

**Directions:**

Preheat oven 350° degrees.

Combine all dry ingredients in a medium bowl and stir until combined.

In a separate medium bowl combine all wet ingredients mix well.

Add wet ingredients to the dry ingredients, mix well without over-mixing, gently fold in blueberries.

In a greased muffin pan, fill batter 3/4 of the way and bake for 25-38 minutes.

Eat warm or room temperature.

Enjoy!

**Preparation time:15 minutes**

**Total time:25-38 minutes**

**Makes:12 servings**

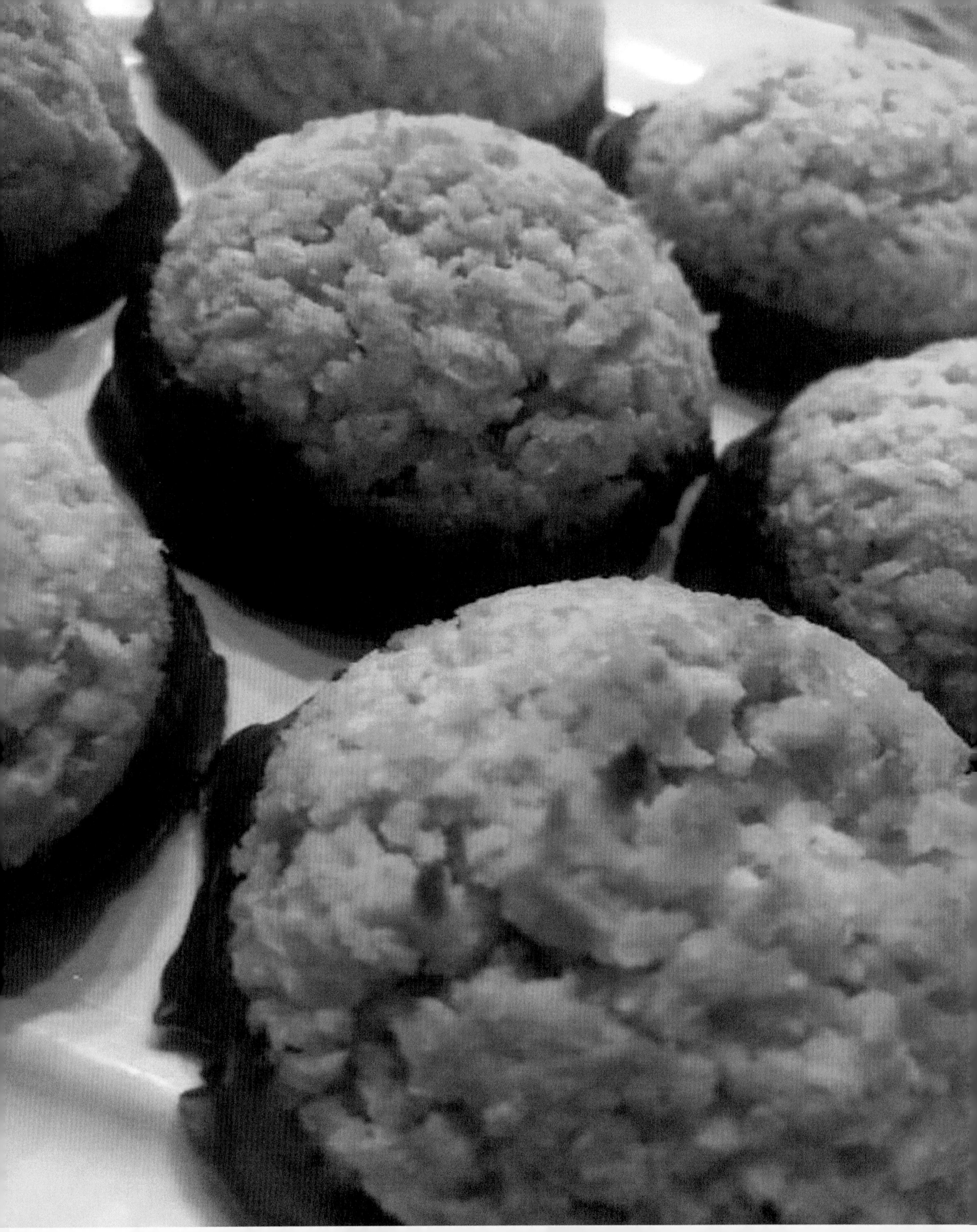

# Chocolate Bottom Pecan Coconut Macaroons

**Ingredients:**

1 cup cane sugar or Monk fruit sweetener

1/2 cup coconut milk

1 tsp kosher salt

2 1/2 tbsp maple syrup

2 tsp vanilla extract

3 cup coconut shreds (unsweetened)

1 1/2 cup all-purpose flour (unbleached)

1 1/2 cup semi chocolate chips

1 1/2 cup chopped pecans

**Directions:**

Preheat the oven 375° degrees.

In a medium bowl add combine all the dry ingredients including the shred coconuts, pecans, and chocolate chips, mix until combined. Add vanilla extract, coconut milk, maple syrup, salt, and monk fruit sweetener or cane sugar.

Next using a 1/4 cup measure, spoon out the mixture and place onto a parchment lined baking sheet.

Bake 18-20 minutes or until golden brown on top. Place baked macaroons on baking rack and let cool completely.

Melt chocolate chips over a double boiler. Dip the cooled macaroons in the melted chocolate covering the bottom portion of the macaroons only. Place macaroons on a parchment lined baking sheet and store in the refrigerator for at least 45-60 minutes or until chocolate is set.

Enjoy!

**Preparation time:15 minutes**

**Total time:18-20 minutes**

**Makes:8 servings**

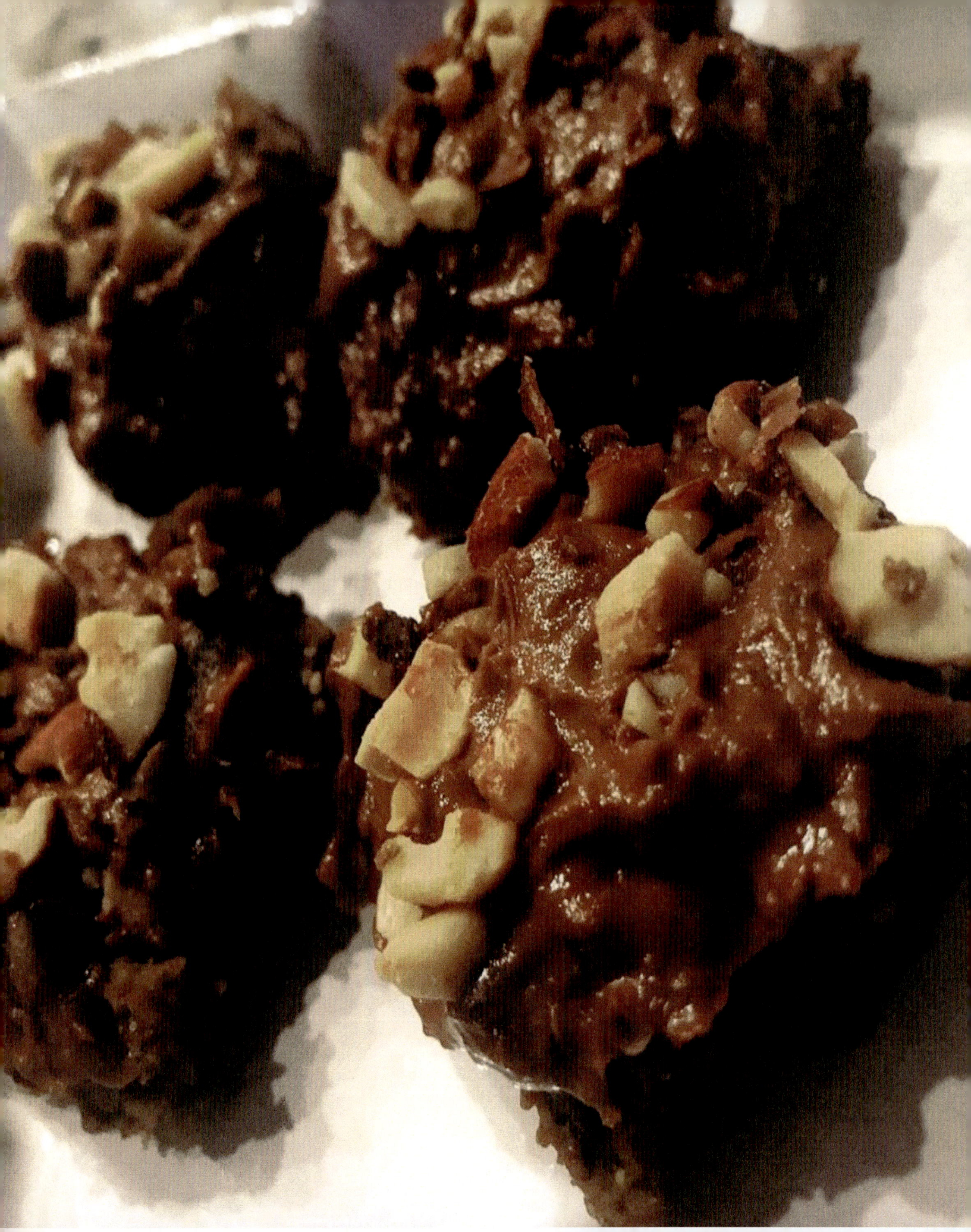

# Vegan Sweet Potato Brownies with Walnuts

**Ingredients:**

1 cup pureed sweet potato (1 15 oz can, or oven roasted)

1/2 cup chickpea (drained & rinsed)

1/2 cup peanut butter

1/4 cup almond flour

1/4 cup cacao powder

1/2 cup maple syrup

1 tsp vanilla extract

1/4 tsp baking powder

1/4 tsp baking soda

1/2 cup semi vegan chocolate chips

1 cup chopped walnuts

**Frosting:**

1 cup pitted Medjool dates

1/2 cup almond butter

¼ cup cocoa powder

½ cup water

**Directions**

Preheat oven to 325 degrees F.

Add all the ingredients except the chocolate chips into a food processor. Blend until completely smooth.

Gently fold in chocolate chips and 1/2 cup walnuts without over-mixing. Pour the mixture into a baking dish (8x8).

Bake for about 25-30 minutes or until they are done (check brownies with a toothpick if brownie mixture is on toothpick continue to bake). Let completely cool before adding the frosting.

Add all frosting ingredients in the food processor mix until completely blend.

Add frost and the remaining walnuts on top of the frosting. Do not play it safe with the frosting.

**Preparation time:15 minutes**

**Total time:30 minutes**

**Makes:6 servings**

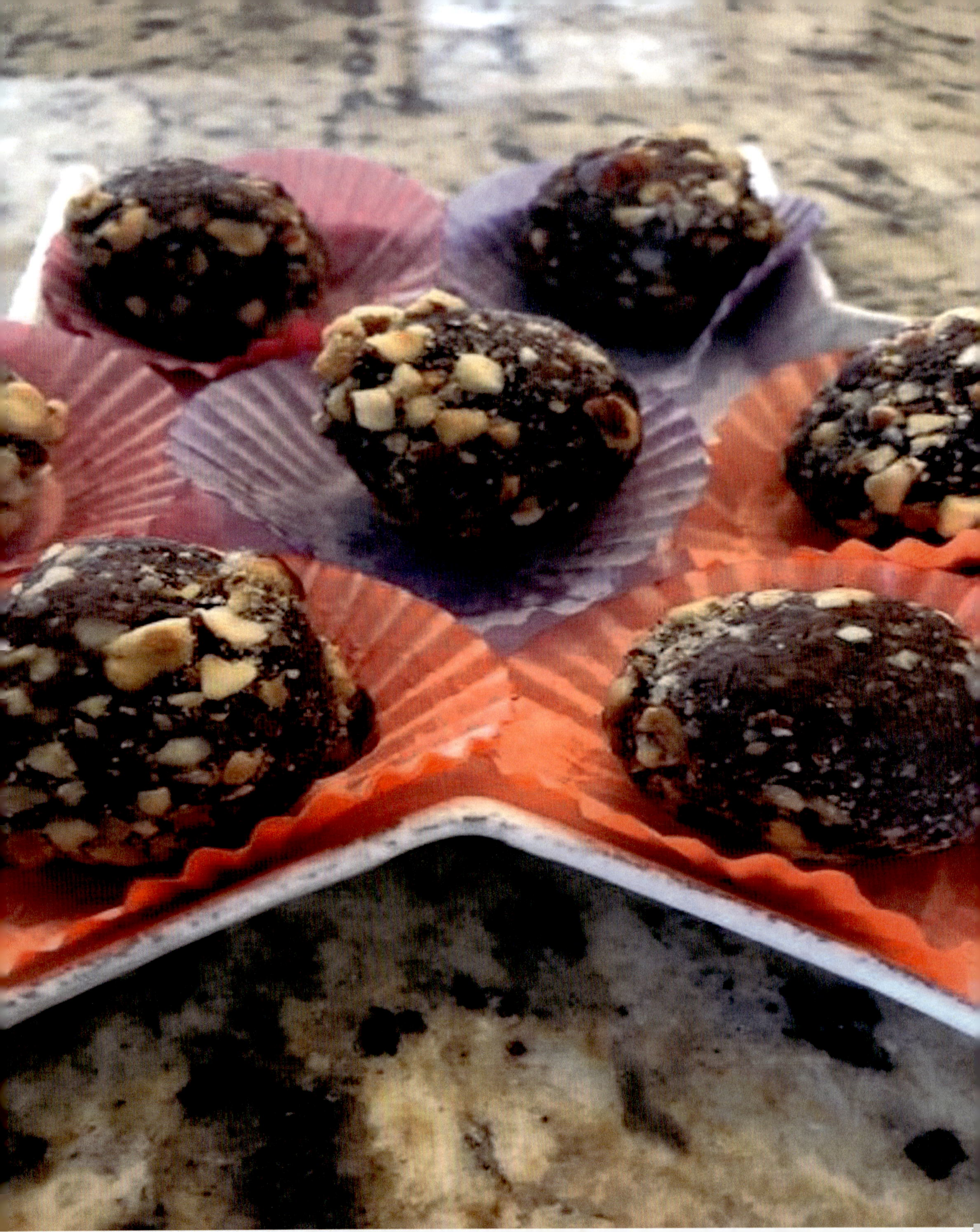

# Vegan Hazelnut Ferrero Rocher

**Ingredients:**

1 1/2 cup vegan semi chocolate chips or chucks

1/2 cup coconut cream

2 tbsp coconut milk

1/2 cup DIY hazelnut butter (hazelnut butter in a jar)

1 1/2 cup roasted hazelnut (1 whole

plus 1/2 chopped)

**Directions:**

In a double boiler add the chocolate chips melt until smooth. Add the coconut cream, coconut milk and hazelnut butter. Mix until smooth. Place mixture in refrigerator for about 2-3 hours or until solid.

Next using the solid mixture scoop a spoon full and roll in your hands forming a small ball. Taking a whole hazelnut press into the center of the ball. Finally, roll ball in the chopped hazelnut, coating the ball completely.

Place the balls on a tray and refrigerator for about 25-30 minutes.

Enjoy one Vegan Hazelnut Ferrero Rocher at a time!

**Preparation time:30 minutes**

**Total time:2hrs 30 minutes**

**Makes:16 servings**

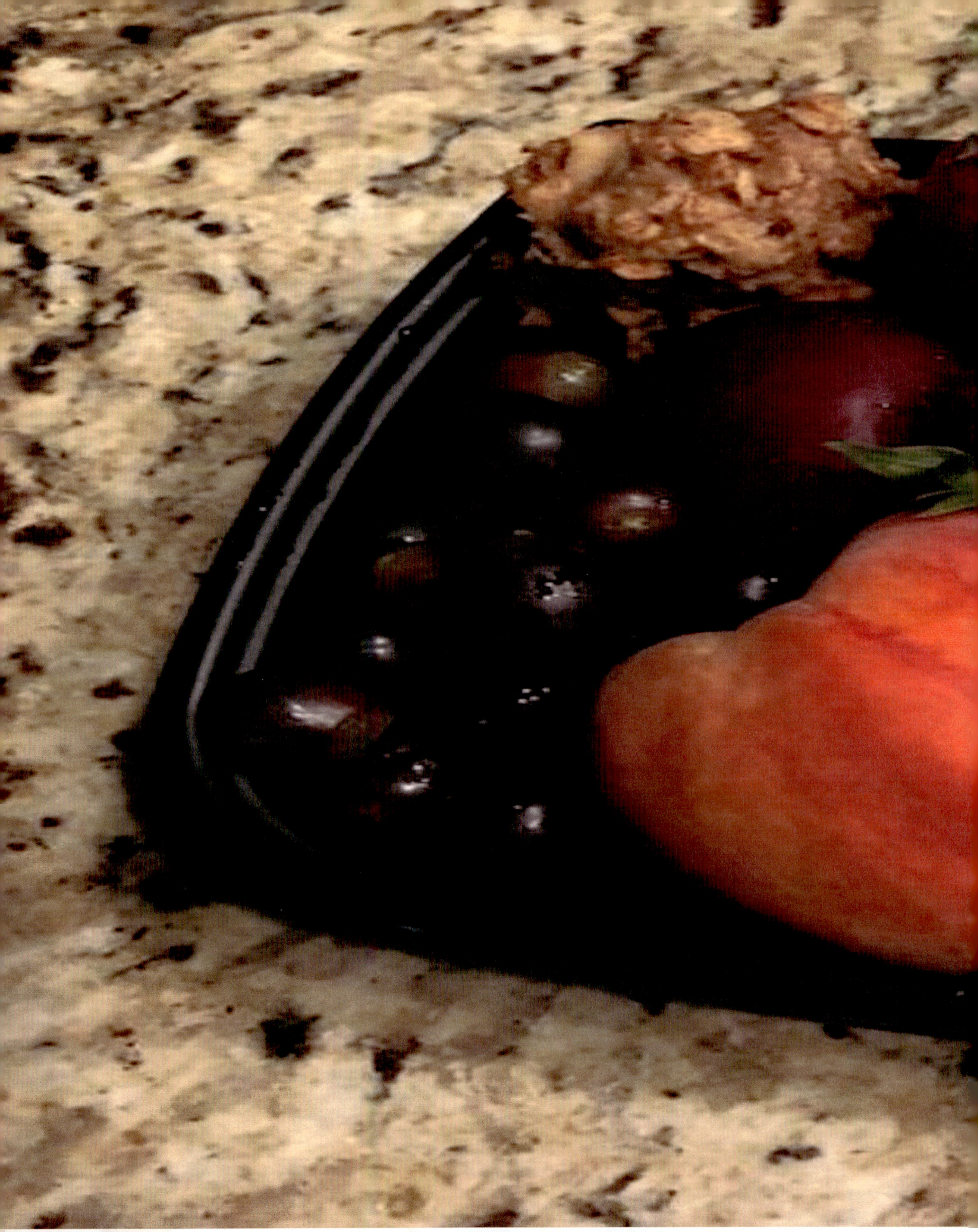

# SMOOTHIES

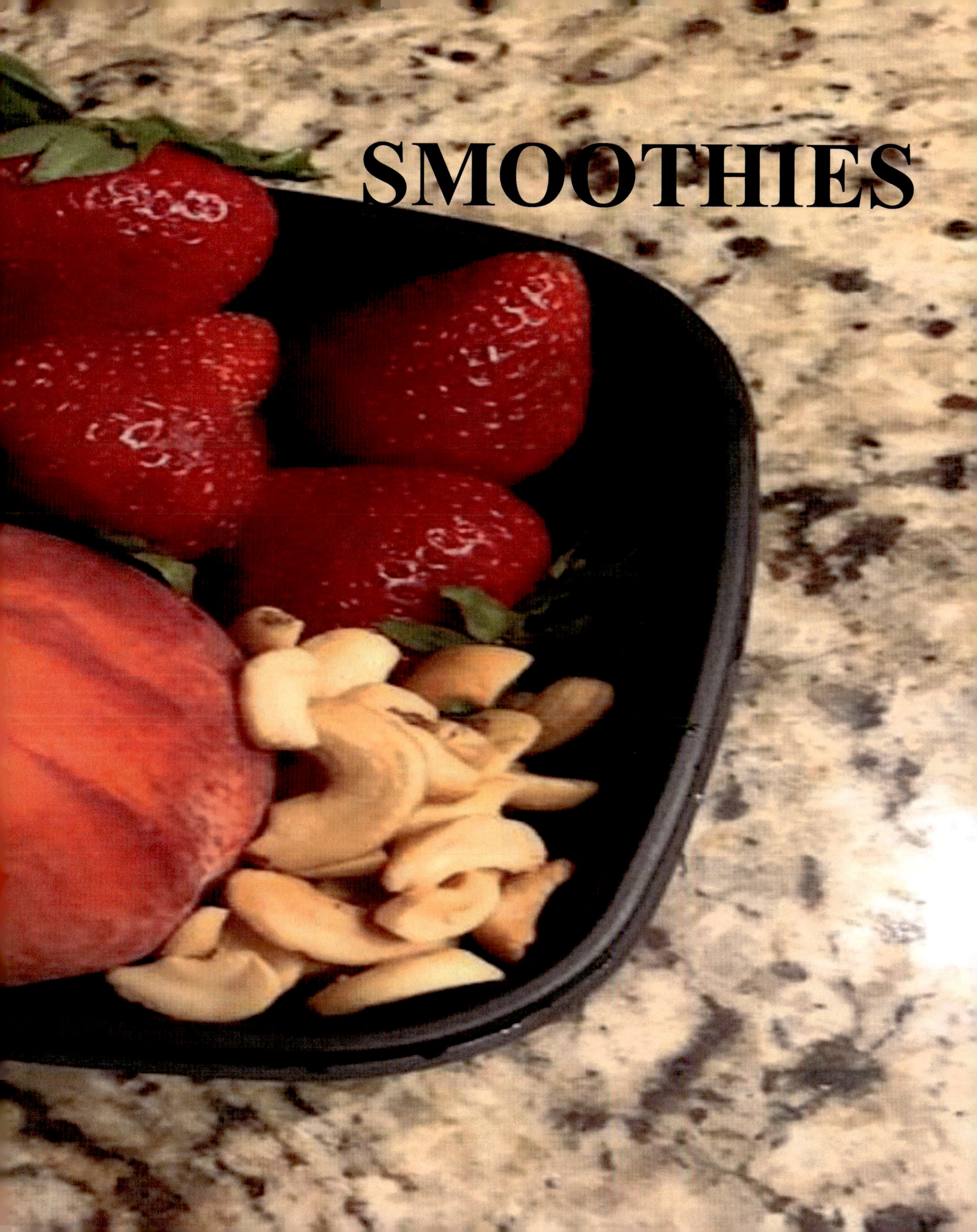

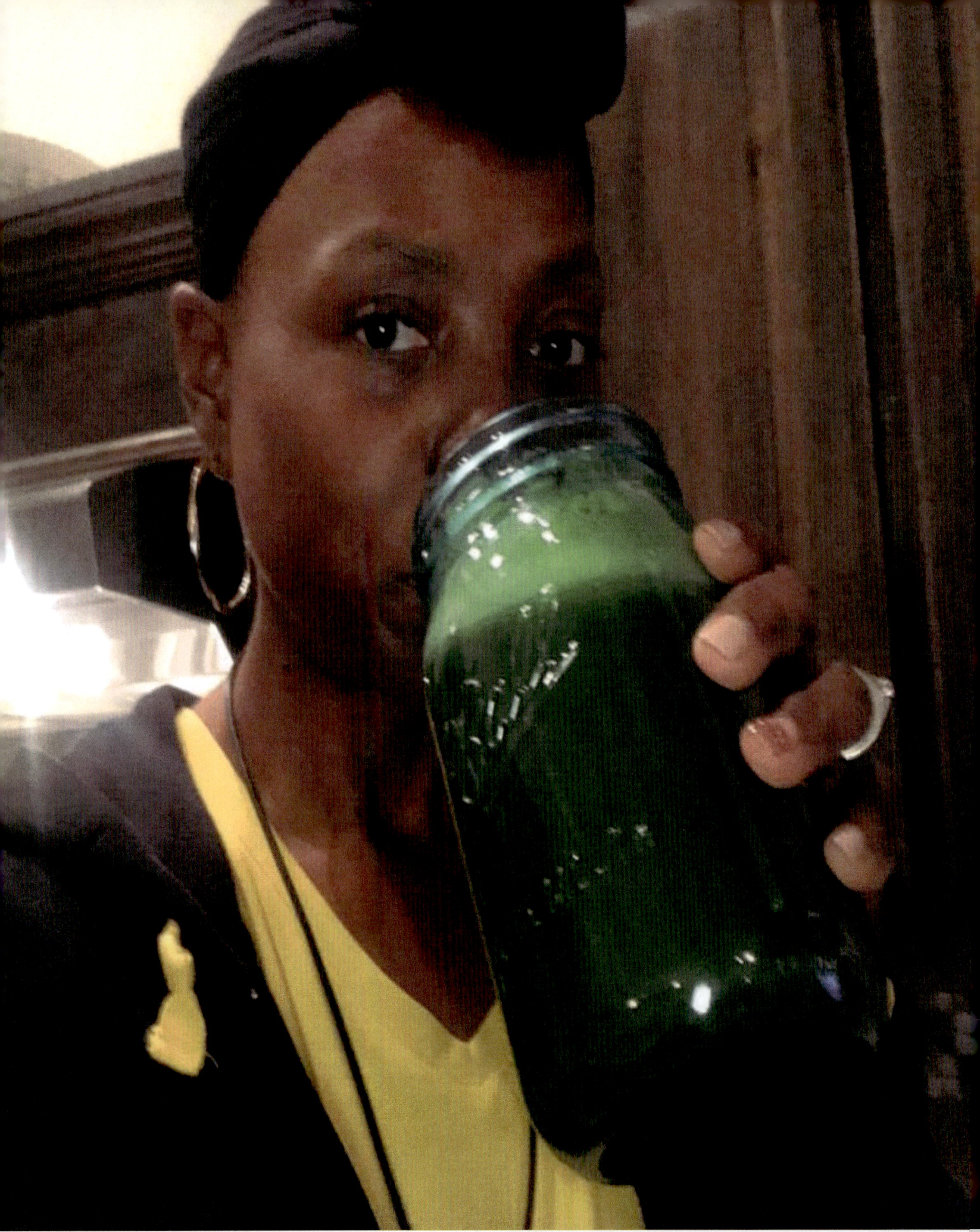

# Truly Green Goodness Raw Juice

10 stalks of kale

5 small red apples (cut in quarters)

1 tbsp of ginger

Combine in juicer and enjoy!

**Makes: 2 servings**

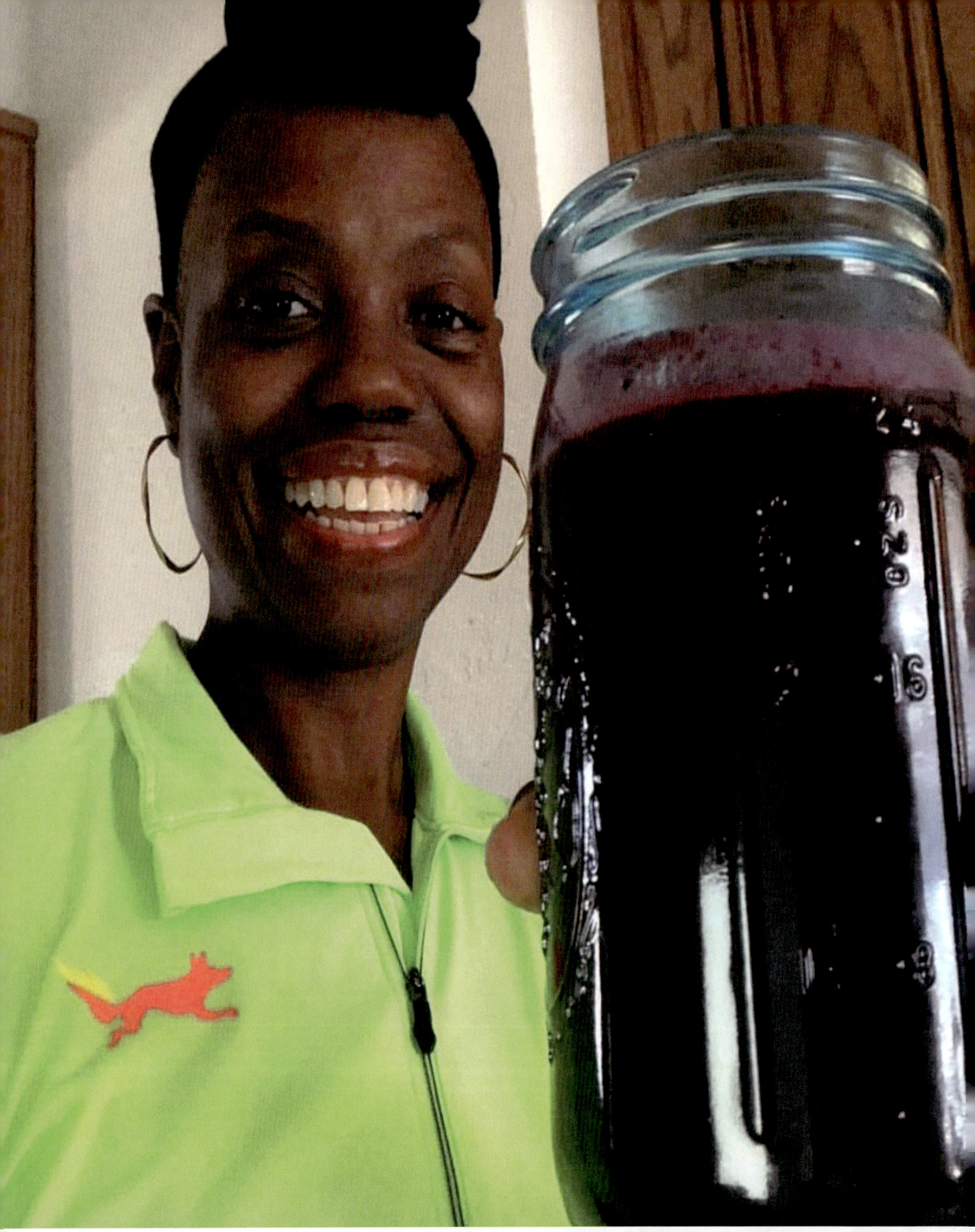

# You Got Me Beat Juice

2 medium beets (cut in half)

1 cup blackberries

1 cup blueberries

1 cup strawberries

1 cup raspberries

5 red apples (cut in half)

Combine in juicer and enjoy!

**Makes: 2 servings**

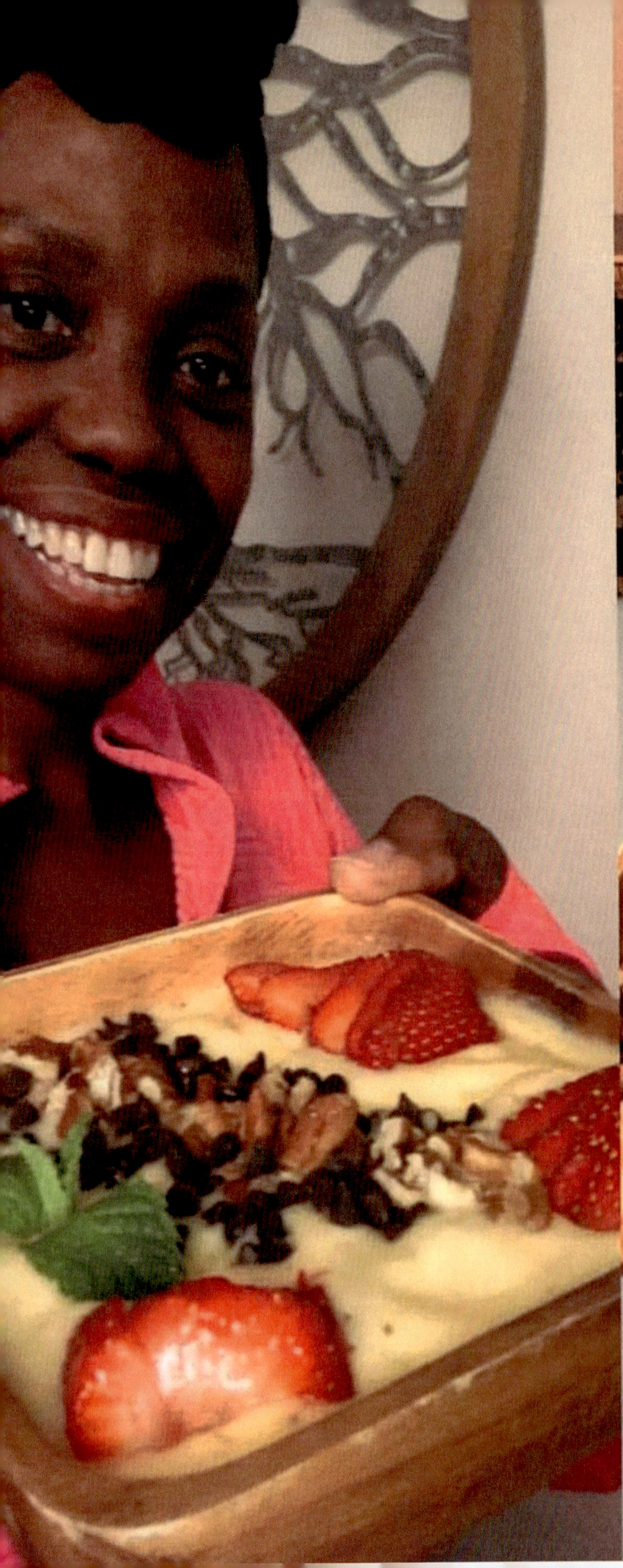

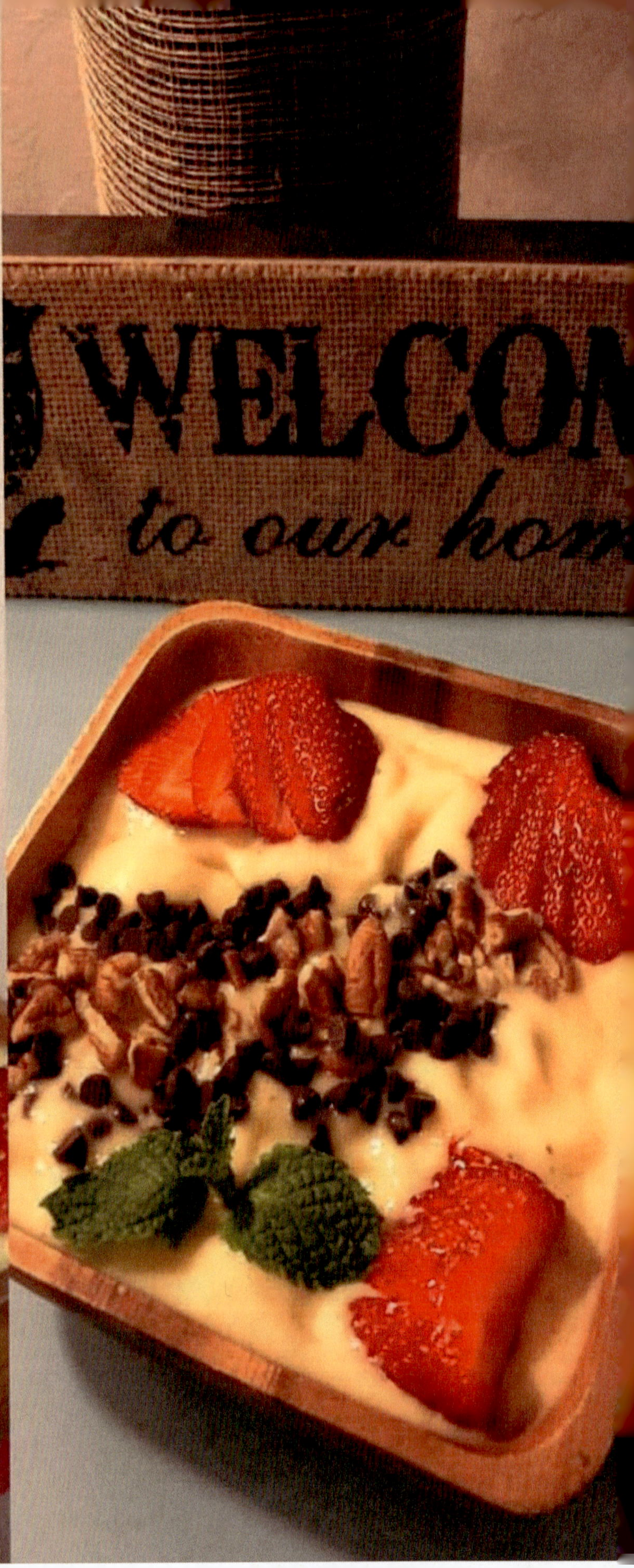
WELCOM
to our hom

# So Right Bright Smoothie Bowl

1 cup mango

1 cup bananas

1 cup peaches

1 cup almond milk

(Make sure your fruit is frozen)

Combine in blender and enjoy

**Makes: 3 servings**

## *Queen for Queen*

*We will not settle for less.*

*We will always give our best.*

*We stand in our black power as black queens*
*changing our communities.*

*Queens, we are more powerful together than apart.*

*Queens take your rightful throne, because you will*
*never stand alone.*

*We will always straighten another queens crown*
*never putting her down.*

*We breathe and speak queendom.*

*Queendom is in our blood its part of our DNA.*

*She has a black king that compliments and address*
*her as black queen and not bi....*

*No let that resonate and penetrate some sh....*

*We keep our head wrapped, held high and our*
*knowledge higher.*

*We are loyal to our true black history and don't*
*accept mediocrity or diversity.*

*We are black queens that demand respect.*

*Our ancestors made sure of that.*

*Queen for Queen*

***Poetically Vegan***

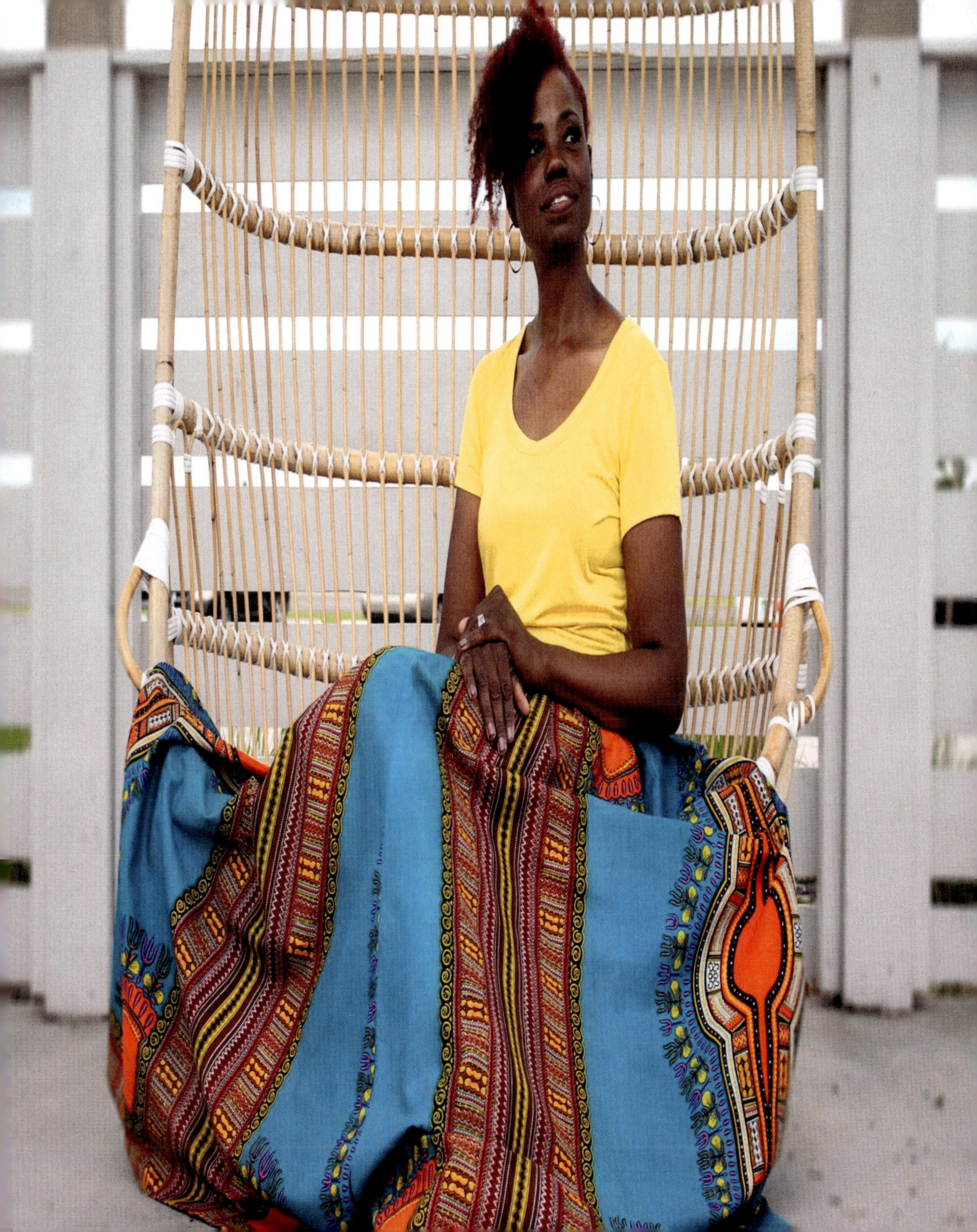

***Roses***

*As the rose petals falls to the ground each day.*

*I will remember and never forget how you made me smile each morning as I leave for work.*

*Your vibrant color brightens my day and leaves an everlasting imprint on my heart.*

*I will not take for granted what you represent, nor will I forget how you smell each day leaving that unique aroma.*

*Roses*

***Poetically Vegan***

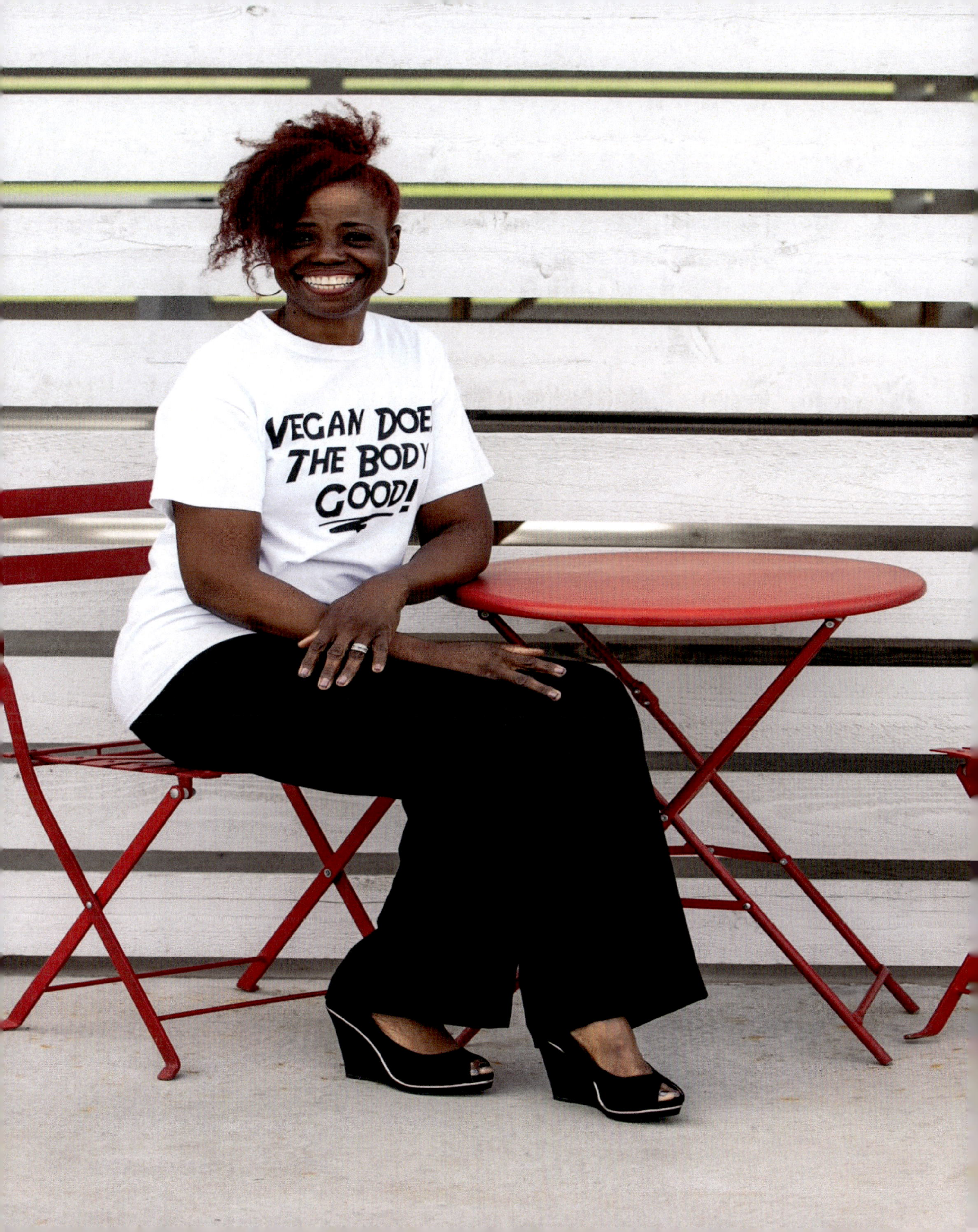
VEGAN DOES
THE BODY
GOOD!

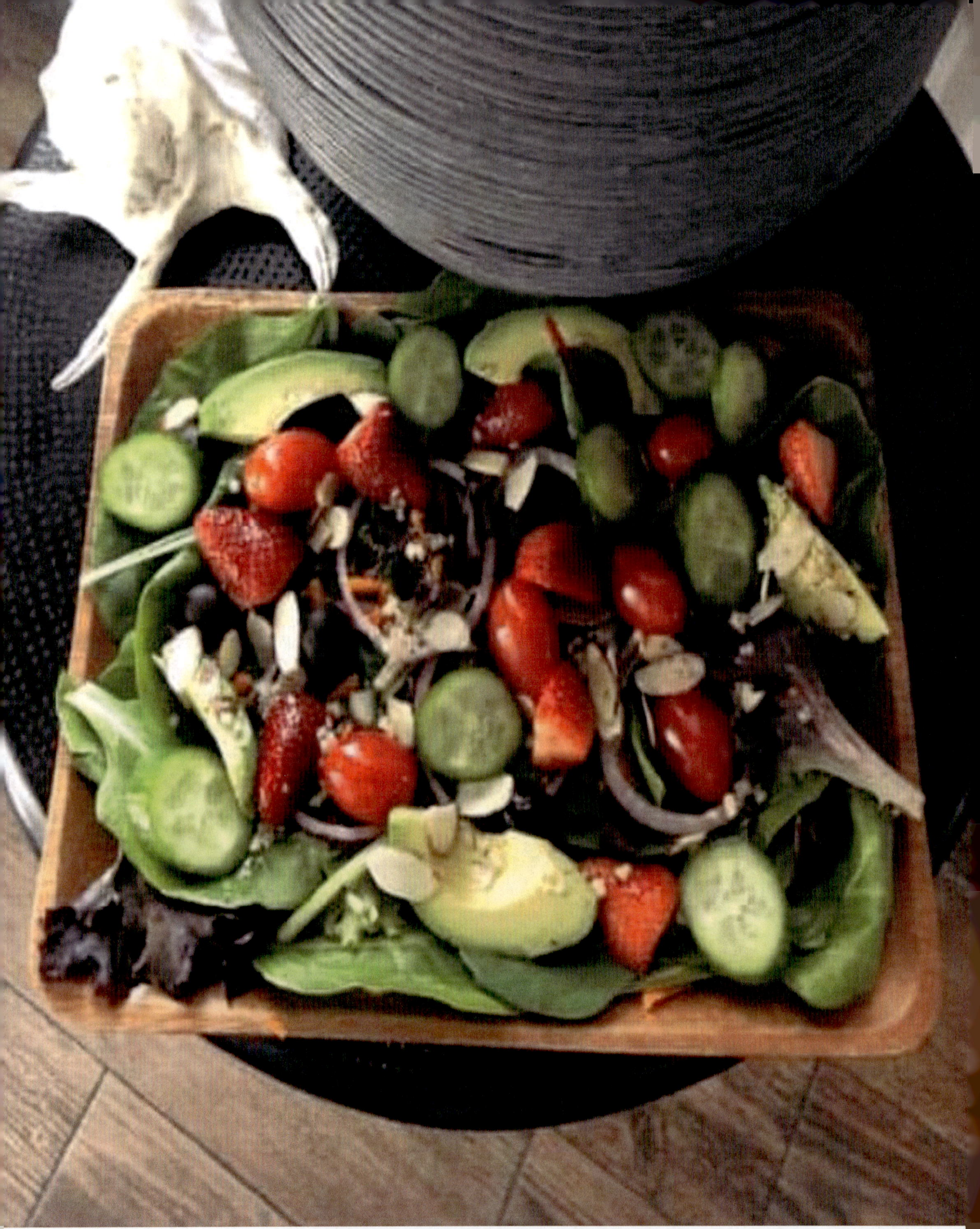

# Gimme All You Got Raw Salad

1 cup mixed greens

1 cup cherry tomatoes

1/2 cup baby cucumbers sliced

1/2 strawberries sliced

1/2 black olives

1/2 shredded carrots

1/2 cup red onions sliced thin

1/2 avocado cut in quarters

1/2 cup sliced almonds

Vegan dressing (your favorite brand)

Combine all ingredients and enjoy!

**Makes: 4 servings**

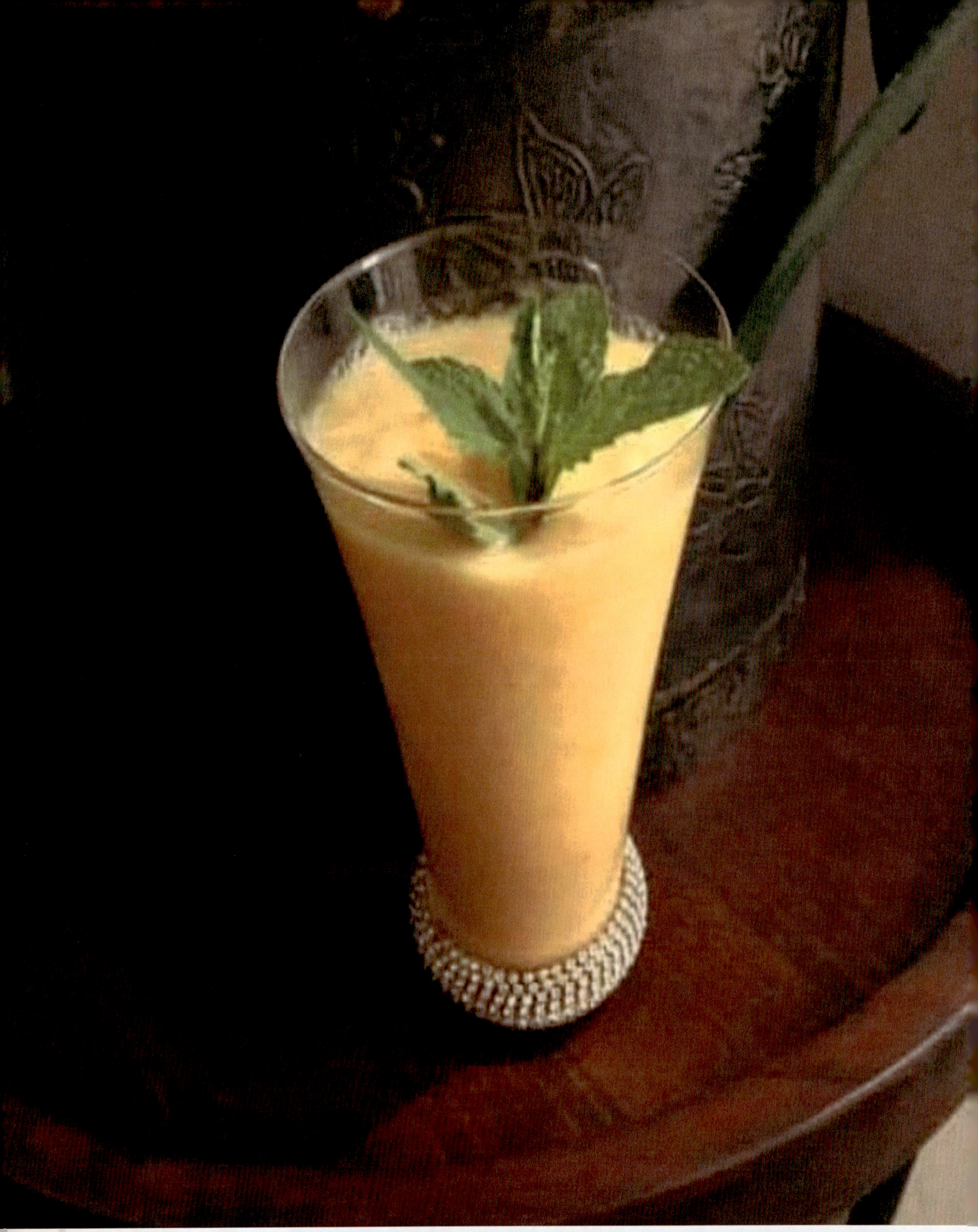

# Pa Ma Pi Smoothie

1 cup papaya

1 cup mango

1 cup pineapple

1 cup almond milk

(Make sure your fruit is frozen)

Combine in blender and enjoy!

**Makes: 2 servings**

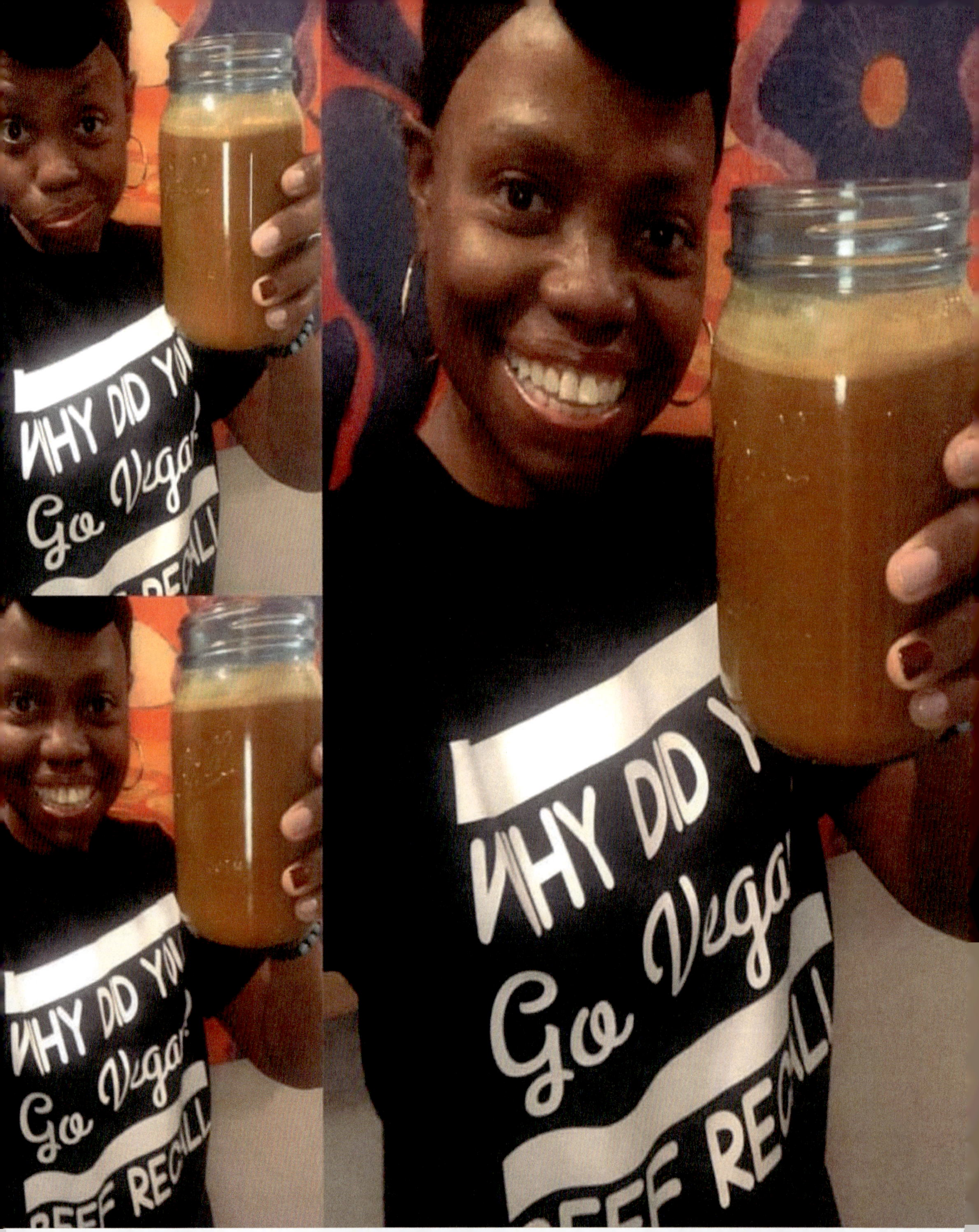

# Carry Me Away Raw Juice

10 whole carrots

6 pink lady apples (cut in half)

4 stacks of celery

Combine in juicer and enjoy!

**Makes: 2 servings**

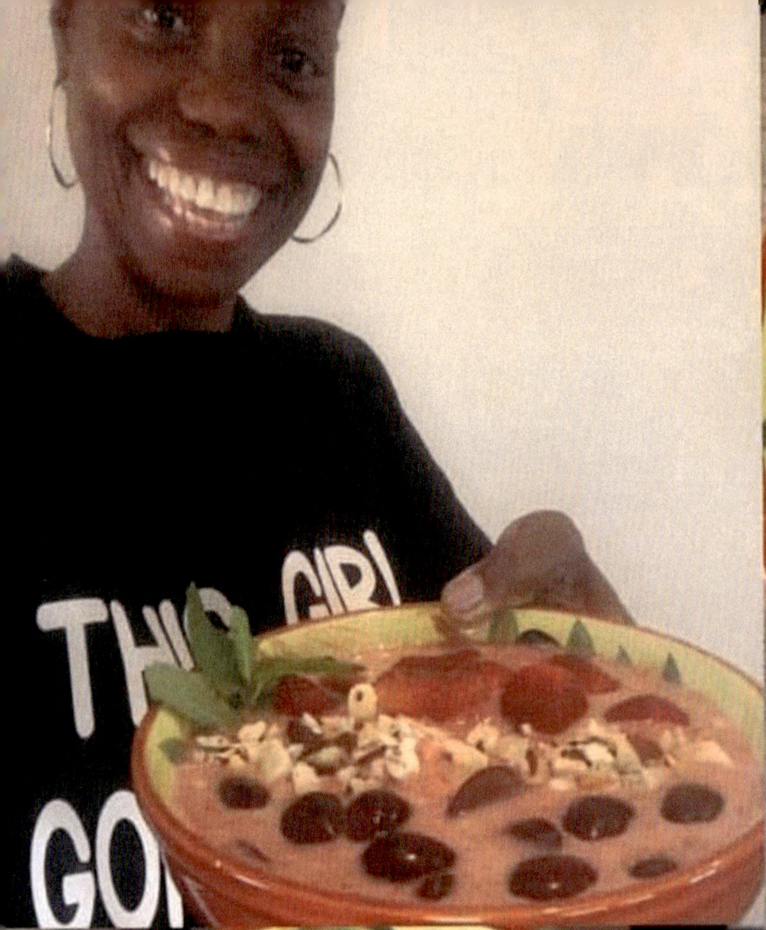
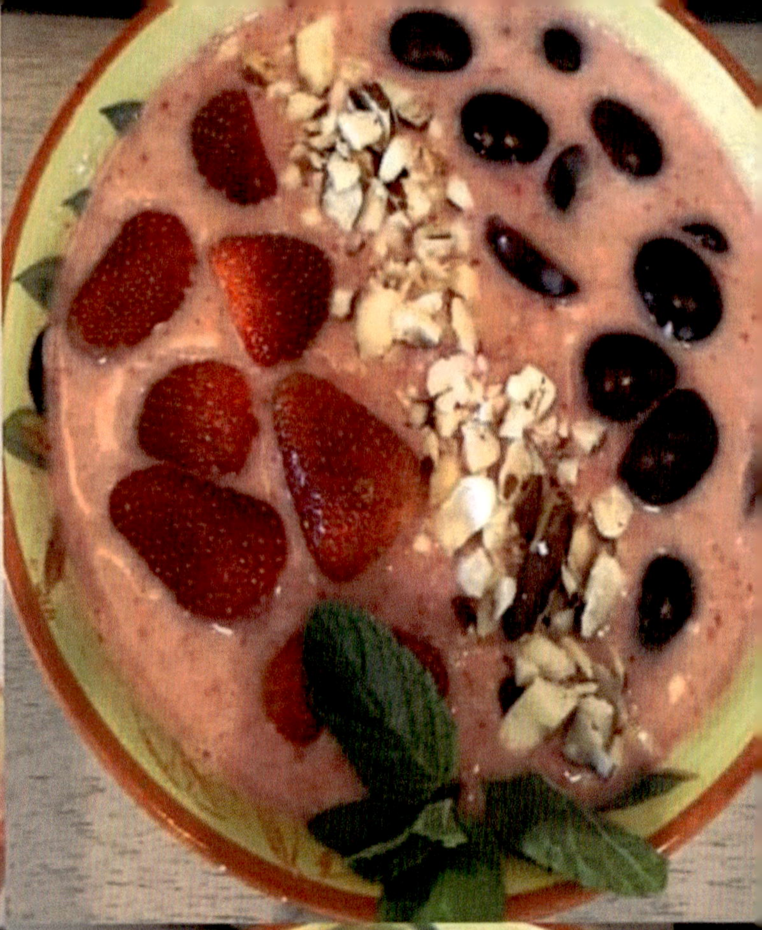
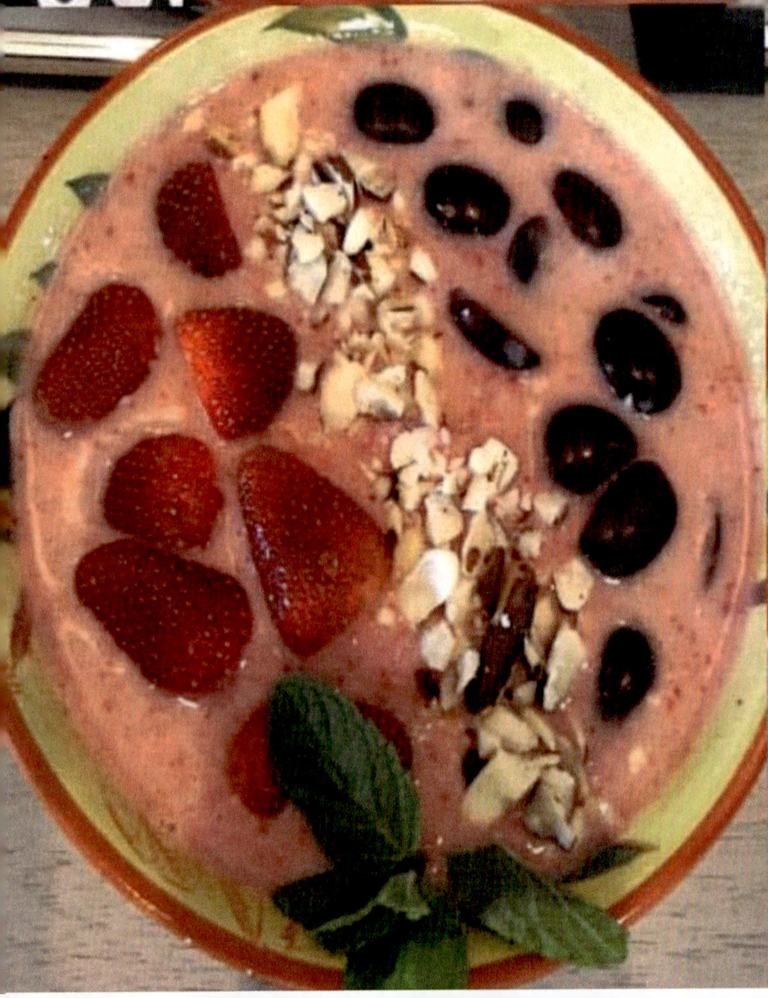
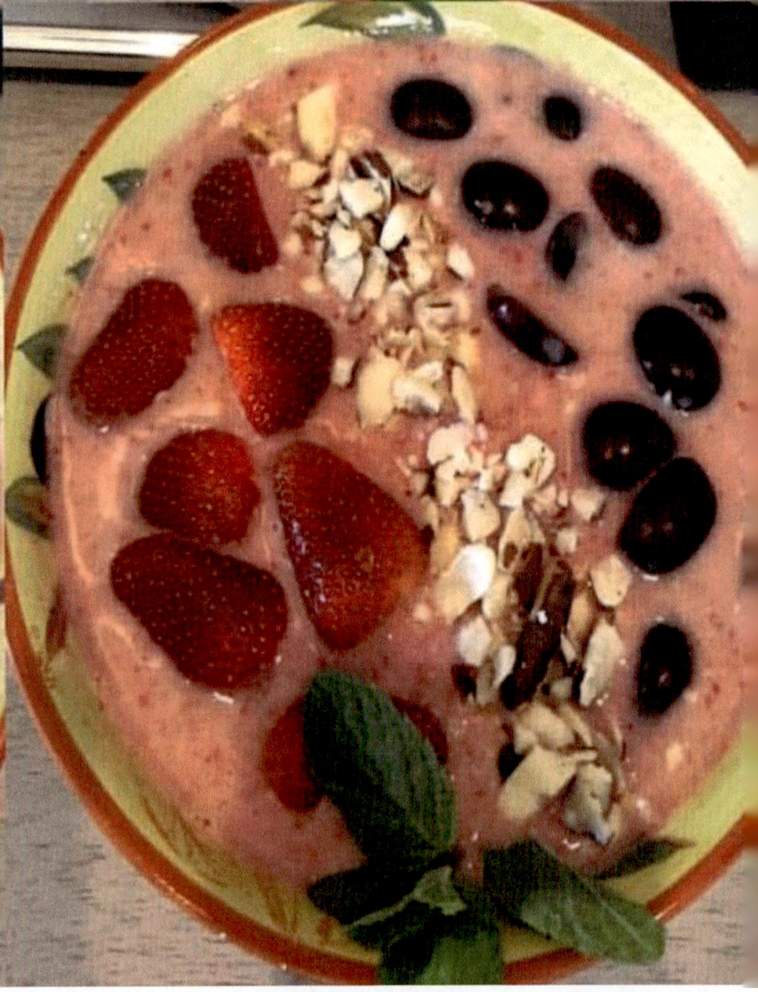

# All In My Bowl Smoothie

8 strawberries

2 bananas (sliced)

1 cup almond milk

Optional: add purple grapes, strawberries & mixed nuts

Make sure your fruit is frozen

Combine in blender and enjoy!

**Makes: 2 servings**

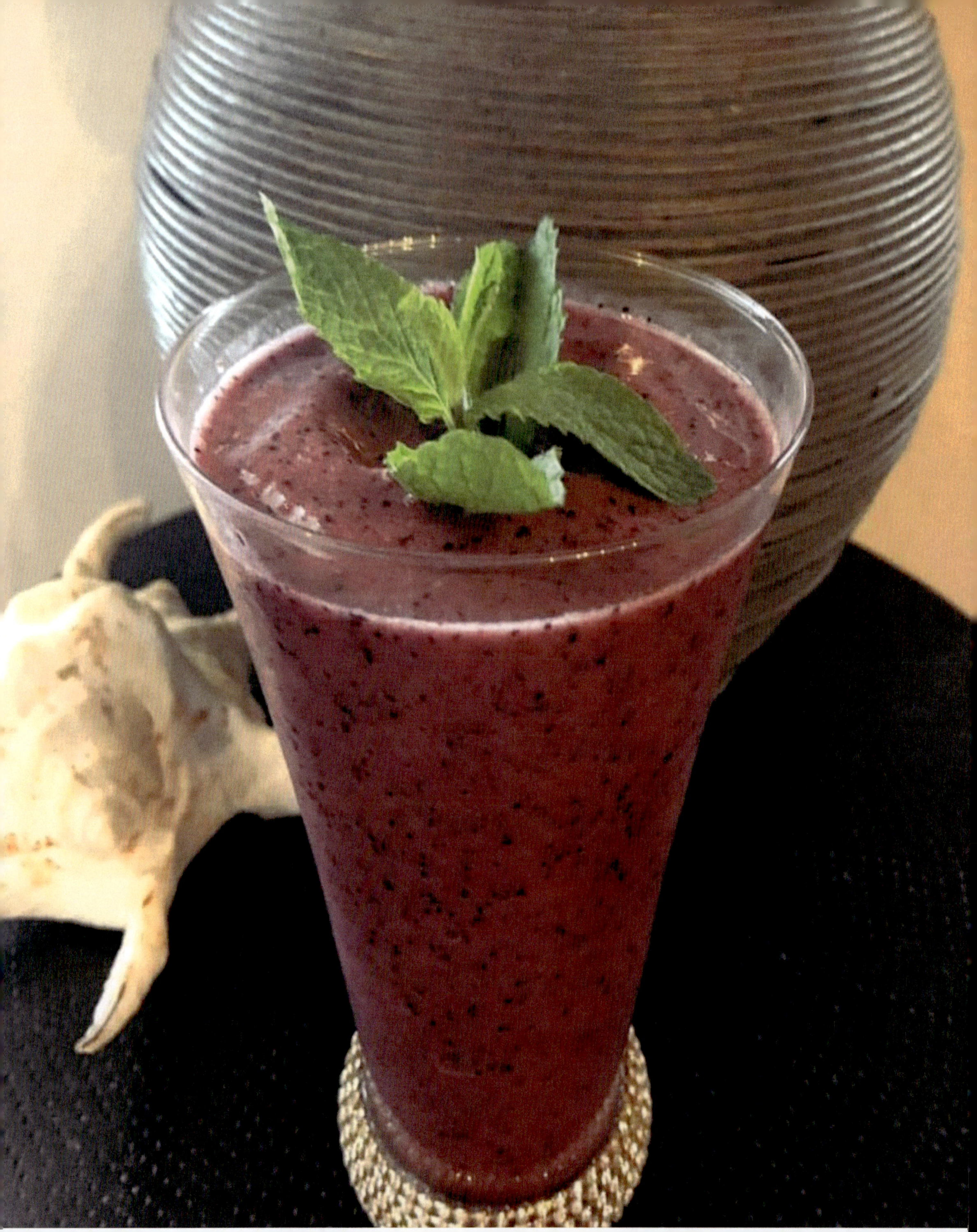

# Blue Moon Smoothie

1 cup blueberries

1 cup banana (sliced)

1 cup almond milk

Make sure your fruit is frozen

Combine in blender and enjoy!

**Makes: 2 servings**

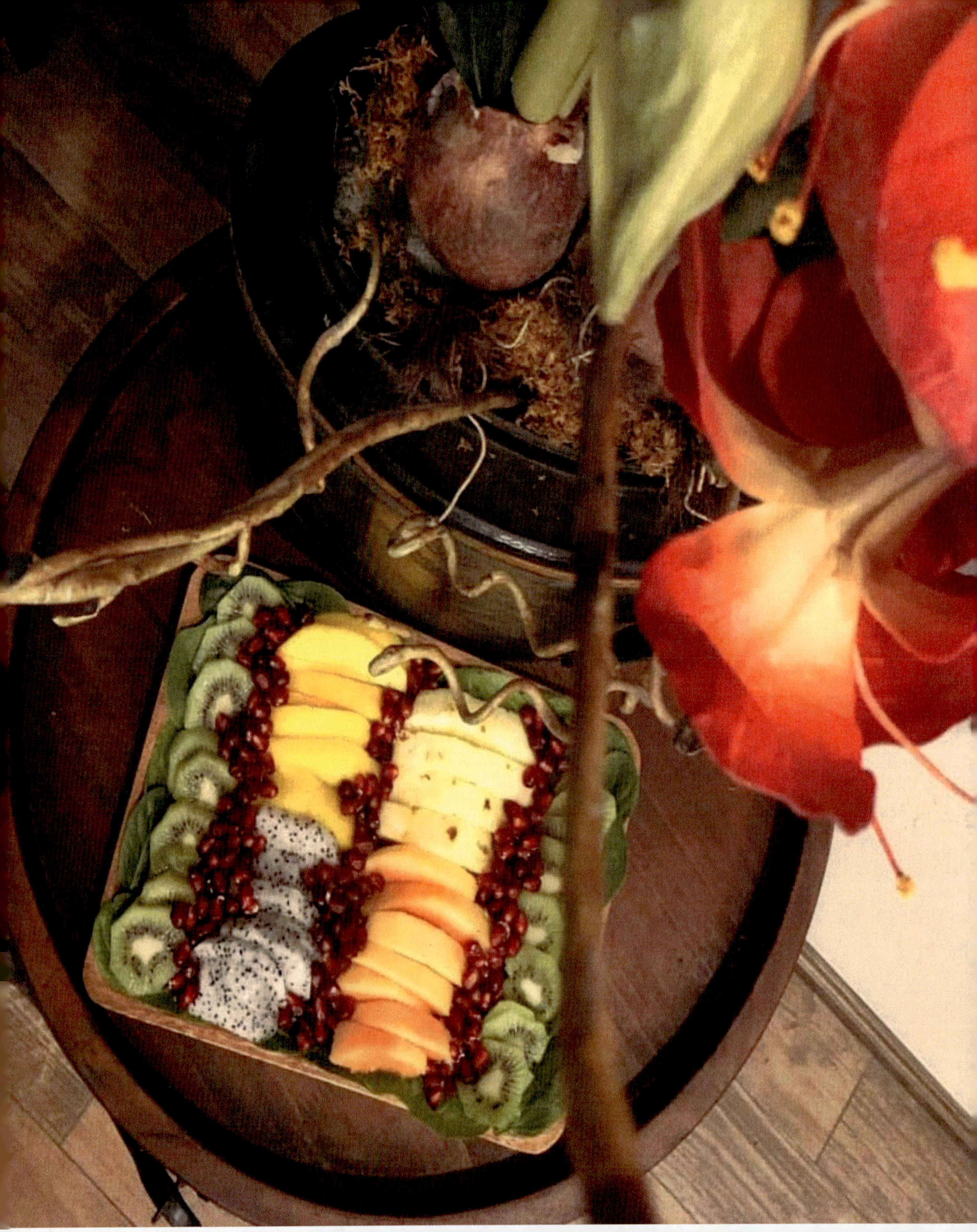

# Pick Off My Fruit Platter

1/2 cup kiwi

1/2 cup mango

1/2 cup passion fruit

1/2 cup pineapples

1/2 cup papaya

1 cup pomegranate (seeded)

Pick what you like and enjoy!

**Makes: 6 servings**

***Negativity***

*I won't let you consume me.*

*I won't let you define me.*

*So, I just say bye and give you a taste of this side eye.*

*See, the vibe you have, the energy you're in, the frequency you spin, I don't want to be in.*

*Hold up, why are you here, oh that's right I let you in because I felt no fear that's why you're here.*

*Your negative touches, your negative thoughts, your negative love, your kisses they don't live here anymore.*

*I walked in your shadows thinking it was the image of me.*

*It was so easy to stay until I found my own way.*

*The vibe you have, the energy you're in, the frequency you spin, I don't want to be in.*

*Negativity*

***Poetically Vegan***

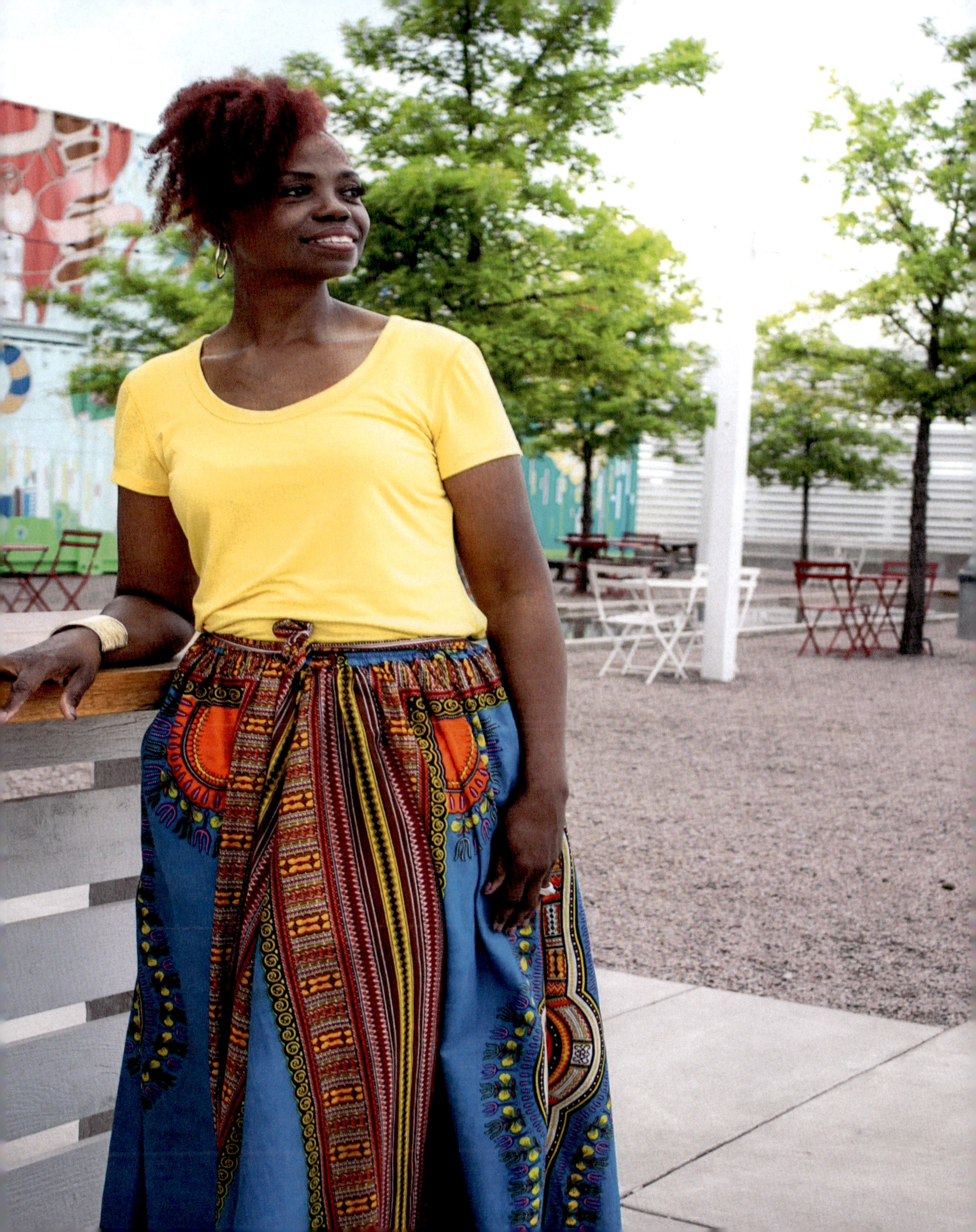

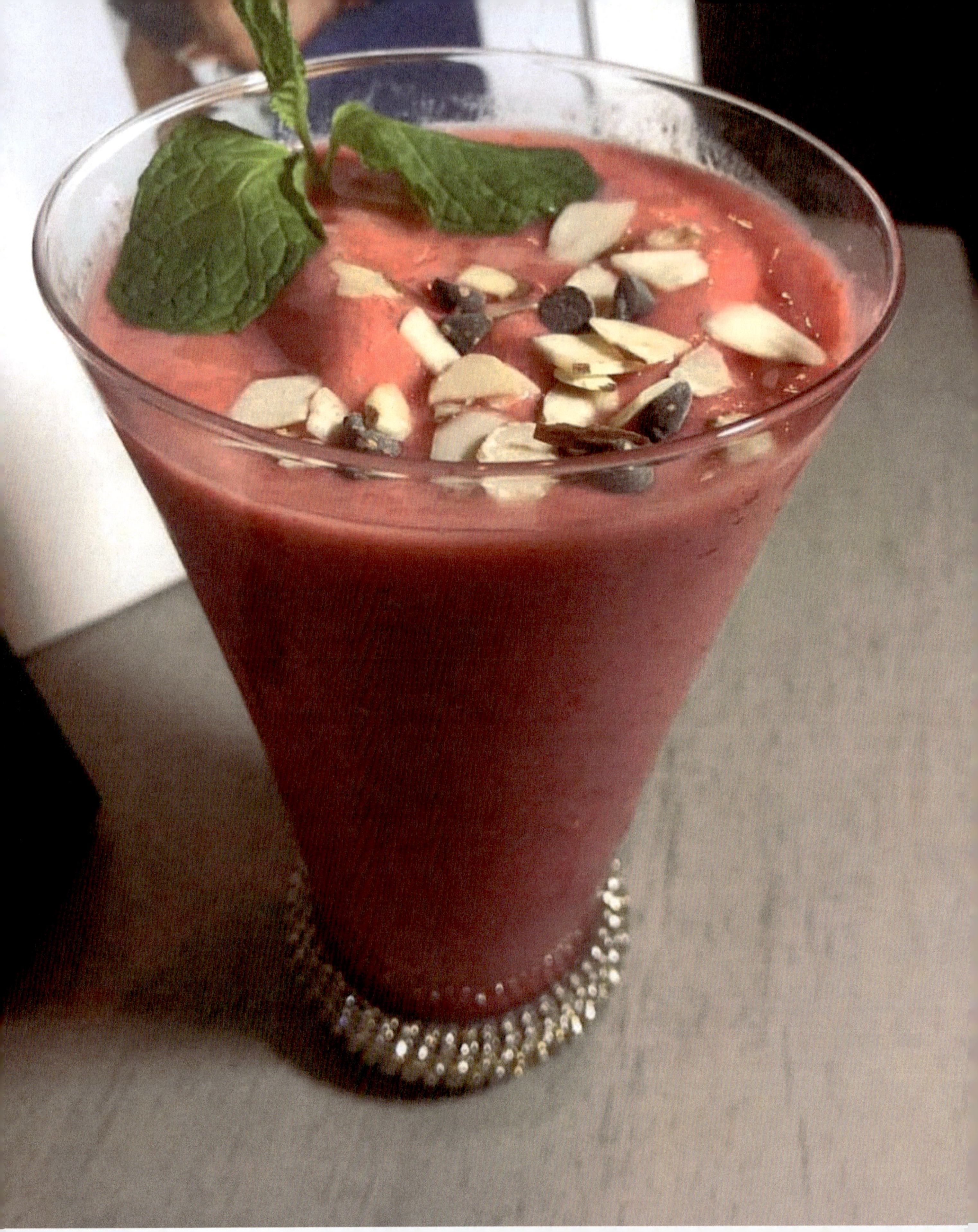

# Raise the Roof Smoothie

1 cup raspberries

1 cup banana (sliced)

1/2 cup almond milk

Make sure your fruit is frozen

Combine in blender and enjoy!

**Makes: 2 servings**

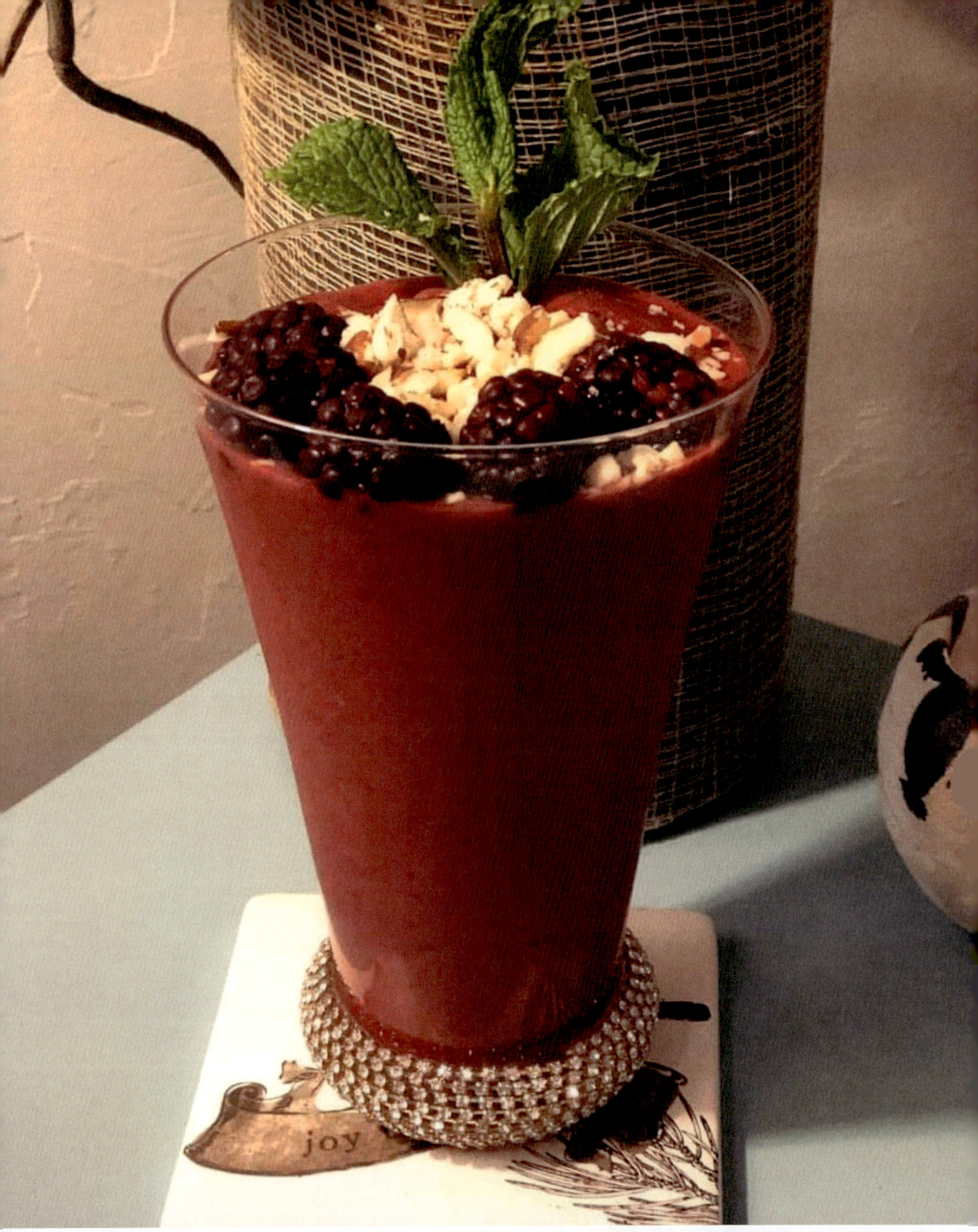
joy

# Don't Hold Back Smoothie

1/2 cup blackberries

1/2 cup banana (sliced)

1/2 cup almond milk

Make sure your fruit is frozen

Combine in blender and enjoy!

**Makes: 2 servings**

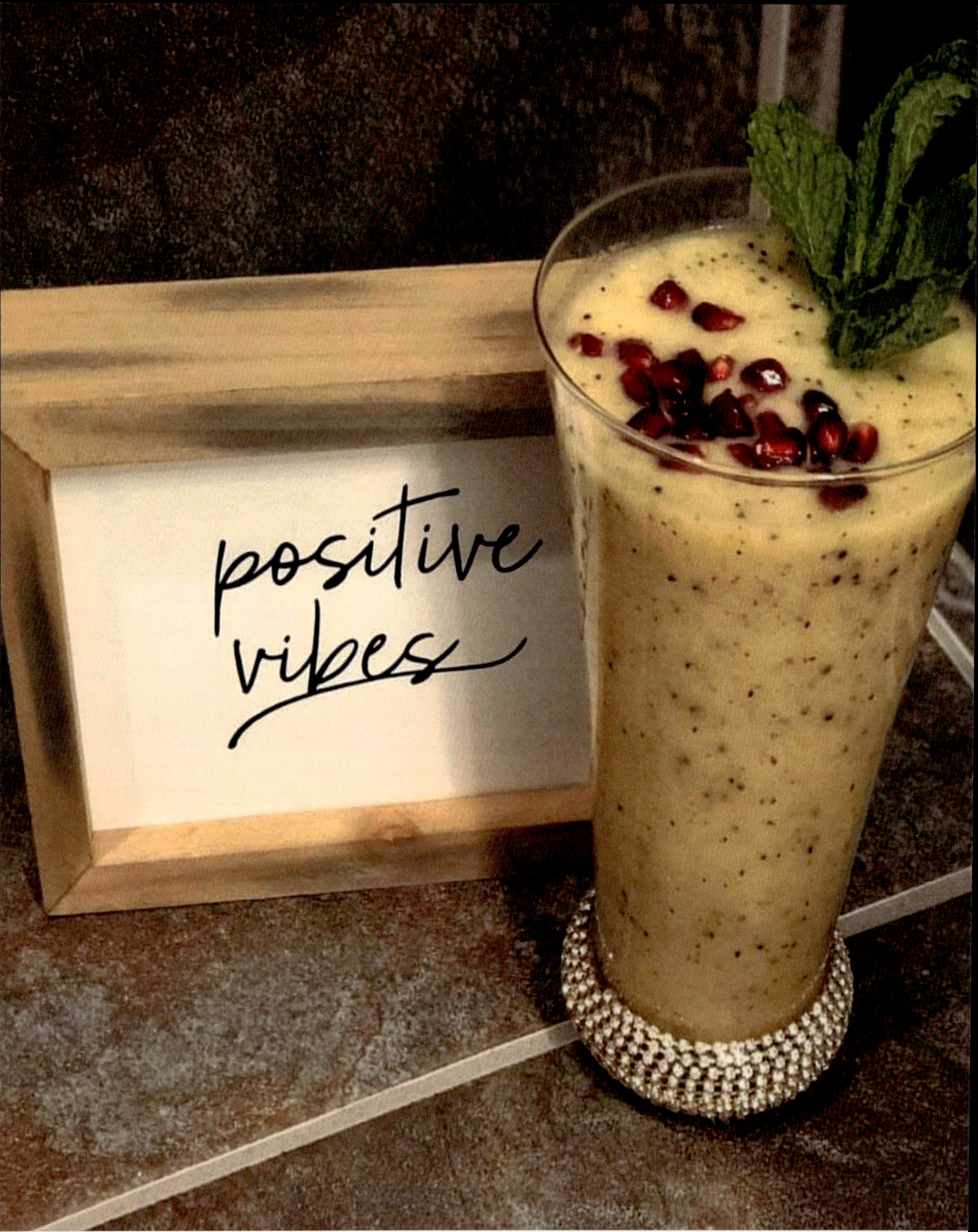
positive
vibes

# Tropical Day Smoothie

1/2 cup mango (sliced)

1/2 cup papaya (sliced)

1/2 cup passion fruit (sliced)

1/2 cup pineapples (sliced)

1/2 cup kiwi (sliced)

1/2 cup almond milk

Make sure your fruit is frozen

Combine in blender and enjoy!

**Makes: 2 servings**

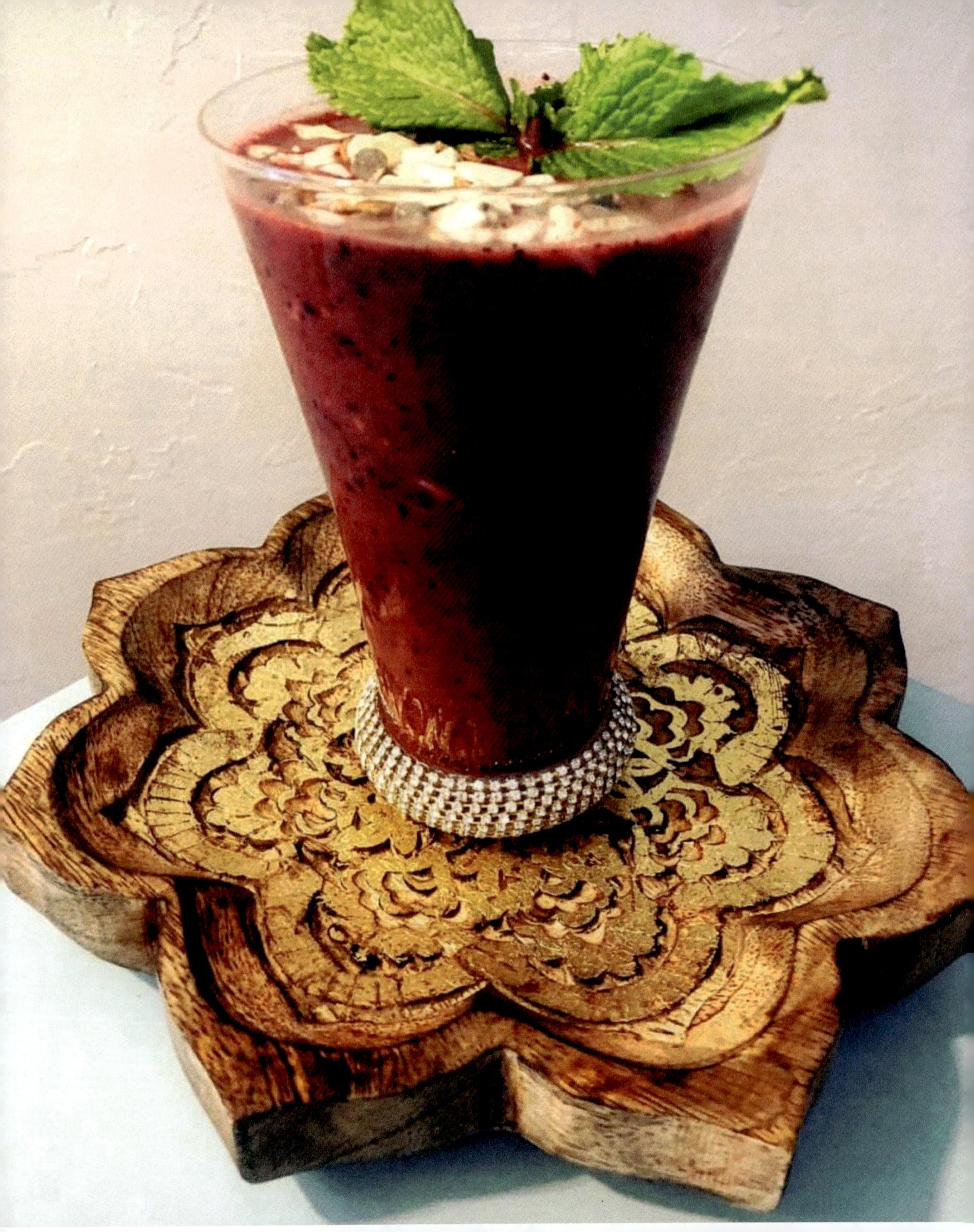

# So Many Berries Smoothie

1/2 cup blueberries

1/2 cup blackberries

1/2 cup bananas (sliced)

1/2 cup almond milk

Make sure your fruit is frozen

Combine in blender and enjoy!

**Makes: 2 servings**

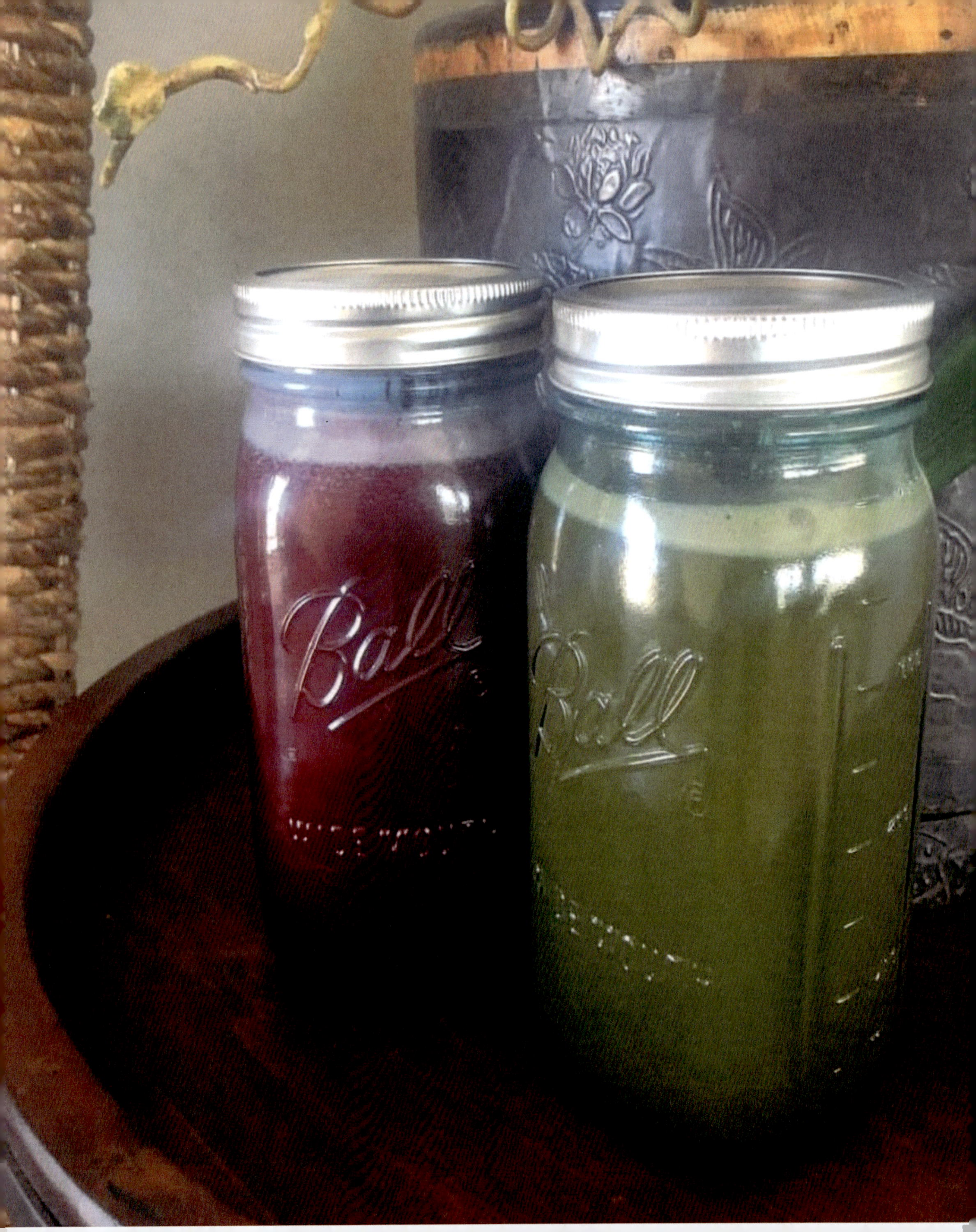
Ball
Ball

# All Day Raw Juice

1 medium beet (cut in half)

1/2 pineapple (cut in half)

4 red apples (cut in quarters)

1 tbsp ginger

5 carrots

4 red apples (cut in quarters)

5 stacks of swiss chard

1 tbsp ginger

Combine in juicer and enjoy!

**Makes: 4 servings**

# APPENDIX

# Handy Tips

# Building Your Pantry

**The first step to building a vegan pantry is to take inventory of what you have. It isn't entirely necessary to have a large pantry filled with tons of ingredients and packaged foods. All you need to do is sit and think about the things that are important to you. Once you figure out what you need and what you're eating preferences are then you can start building things to put in your pantry.**

**Here are some examples of pantry items. Remember this list is just designed to be a starting point.**

**Spices & Herbs: turmeric, nutmeg, ginger, Himalayan salt, black pepper, allspice, paprika, garlic, onion powder, thyme, rosemary, oregano, parsley, dill, curry powder, cayenne pepper, cumin**

**Grain: Whole wheat, brown rice, whole oats, buckwheat, whole grain barley, quinoa, bulgur, wheat rye, freekeh, couscous**

**Pasta: vegetable, chickpea, gluten free, edamame, brown rice, orzo**

**Legumes: chickpea, lentils, peas, kidney beans, black beans, pinto beans, navy beans**

**Nuts & Seeds: sunflower seeds, pumpkin seeds, sesame seeds, fennel seeds, flax seeds, chia seeds, moringa seeds, almonds, walnuts, hazelnuts, cashews, peanuts, pine nuts, pistachios, pecans, brazil, coconuts, macadamia, cocoa beans**

**Oil: avocado oil, coconut oil, grapeseed oil, almond oil, olive oil, safflower oil, sesame oil**

**Vinegar: red, white, champagne, sherry, apple cider vinegar, balsamic, malt**

**Flour: Spelt flour, chickpea flour, wheat flour, rice flour, almond flour, coconut flour, baking flour, vital**

**wheat gluten**

**Sugar: date sugar, coconut sugar, palm sugar, brown sugar, imperial sugar, maple syrup, brown rice syrup, agave syrup, molasses (they have no bone char)**

## Here is a list of some of my favorite powder superfoods to incorporate into your healthy lifestyle regimen.

1. Spirulina:

Iron, protein, calcium, immune-boosting, vitamin A

2. Hemp:

Plant-based protein, fiber, omega 3s, amino-acids, calcium, magnesium, iron

3. Cocoa powder:

Magnesium, fiber, health heart flavonols

4. Maco powder (Peruvian ginseng):

Energy boost, reduce stress, cognitive enhancer, enhance fertility and boost libido, improve stamina, protein, vitamin C, fiber, amino acids

5. Flax seed:

Omega-3 fatty acids, dietary fiber, phytochemicals (lignans)

6. Chia seeds:

Antioxidant, vitamins & minerals, fiber

7. Matcha:

Green tea powder, antioxidant flavonols, increase energy and focus

8. Baobab:

Calcium, fiber, potassium, magnesium, vitamin C, antioxidants

9. Acai:

Antioxidants, vitamins, minerals, amino acids

10. Camu Camu:

Amino acids, vitamin C, phytochemicals, minerals

11. Moringa:

Antioxidants, vitamins and minerals, amino acids

12. Turmeric:

Magnesium, iron, fiber, vitamin B6

13. Chlorella:

Protein, vitamins and minerals, fiber

# Index

## Entrees

Vegan Stuffed Romain Lettuce.........................8
Vegan Stuffed Japanese Sweet Potato................10
Vegan Loaded Nachos.................................12
Macaroni and Cheese BBQ Sandwich................14
Vegan Cabbage Potato Hash...............................16
BBQ Street Tacos..........................................18
Mixed Veggie Pan-Fry..................................20
***I Can and I Will***.........................................22
Vegan Double Cauliflower Baked Yukon Potato....23
Vegan Chickpea Macaroni Chipotle Salad................26
Golden Brown Falafel Burger....................................30
Golden Brown Falafel Balls.......................................32
Double Cauliflower Black Truffle...............................34
I Can't Believe It's Not Chicken Nuggets.....................36
I Can't Believe It's Not a Chicken Sandwich................38
***Reach Deeper***.......................................................40
Vegan Veggie Crumble Salad......................................42
Vegan Veggie Patty w/ Pearl Cous Cous Salad............44
Vegan Veggie Bunless Burger.........................46
Veggie Patty Crumble....................................48
Vegan Thai-Style Buddha Bowl/Plate...................50
Spicy Vegan Calamari...................................52
Roasted Butternut Squash Soup.........................54
Roasted Acorn Squash Wedges..........................56
***Dreams***......................................................58
Stuffed Portobello Mushrooms...........................60

## Desserts

Chocolate Chip Banana Nut Muffins.............................64
Vegan Cashews Chocolate Chip Protein Balls...............66
Apple Carrot Cookies.....................................................68
Vegan Banana Walnut Bread.............................70
Vegan Coconut Chocolate Chip Walnut Squares......72
Vegan Blueberry Coconut Yogurt Muffins............74

Chocolate Bottom Pecan Coconut Macaroons..........76
Vegan Sweet Potato Brownies w/ Walnuts............78
Vegan Hazelnut Ferrero Rocher.........................80

# Smoothies

Truly Green Goodness Raw Juice............................84
You Got Me Beat Juice......................................86
So Right Bright Smoothie Bowl.............................88
***Queen For Queen***..........................................*90*
***Roses***..........................................................*92*
Gimme All You Got Raw Salad..............................94
Pa Ma Pi Smoothie............................................96
Carry Me Away Raw Juice...................................98
All In My Bowl Smoothie....................................100
Blue Moon Smoothie.........................................102
Pick Off My Fruit Platter....................................104
Negativity.......................................................106
Raise The Roof Smoothie...................................108
Don't Hold Back Smoothie..................................110
Tropical Day Smoothie.......................................112
So Many Berries Smoothie..................................114
All Day Raw Juice............................................116

## ***Dedication***

*There's not a day that goes by that I don't think of you and your smile. Thank you for giving me the love of sharing the importance of living a healthy lifestyle.*
*Thank you, Mother, (Grandmother "T") for showing me that healthy living is part of life. I love you and miss you so much.*

*Love,*
*Kaye (my mom always called me Kaye)*

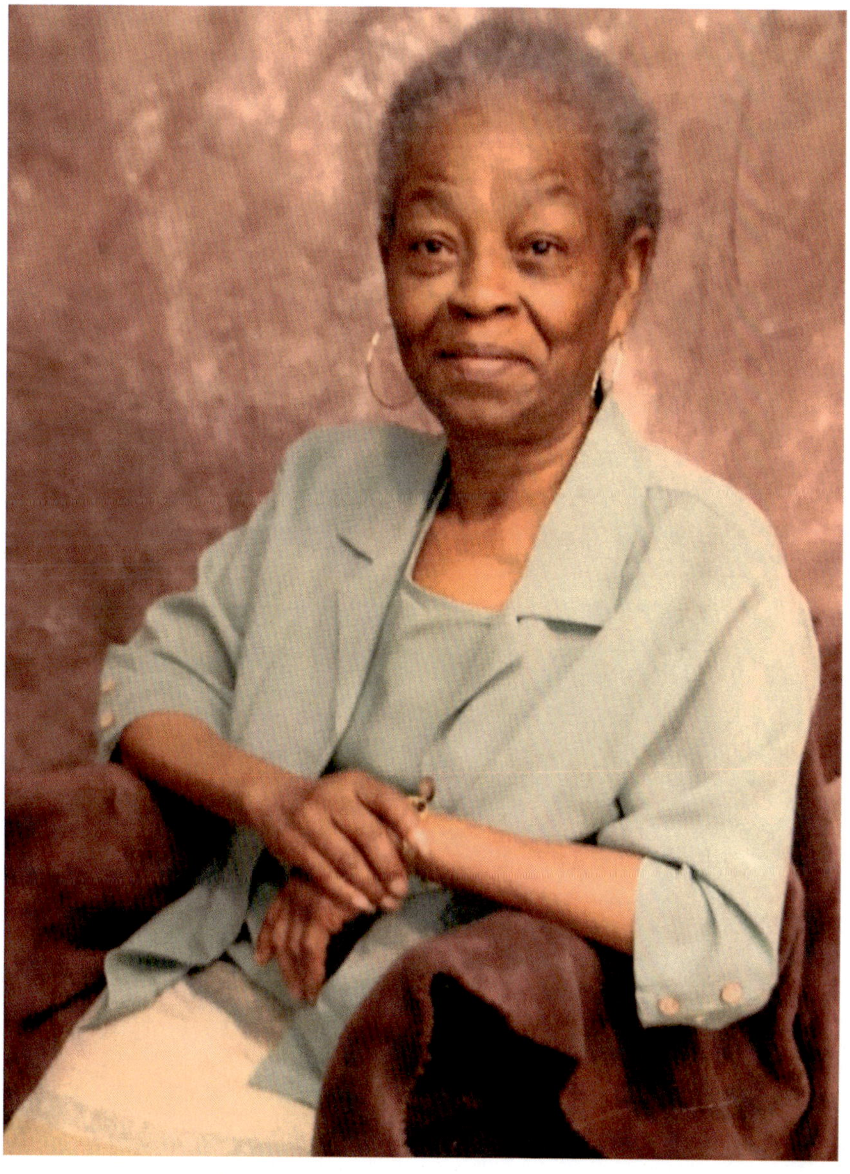

# *Acknowledgements*

Rice Photography OKC
Laney Love Memories
Martin Luther King Jr. (Poem Quote)

## Recipe Reviews

**July 23, 2019**

*"Meal prep yummy thanks Aunt FeFe #veganstyle*" ~ **Markita Shinault-Hardiman**

**August 7, 2019**

"*Meal prep by of course the one and only Felisa Kaye Cargile I gets mine u beta get in on it, cause ya"ll are clearly missing out!!"*~ **Destiny Foster**

**October 28, 2019**

"*Needed some food preps for a road trip and with celiac it makes it harder to find gluten friendly meals. Felisa's veggie patty was amazing! Can't wait to try more*!" ~ **Becki Word**

**October 20, 2019**

*"I went to a party that had Ms. Felisa cater one of her Hispanic vegan dishes and I was blown away! She had everything from the vegan cheese to the vegan sour cream and it all tasted phenomenal! The meal consisted of nachos and soft tacos. She had the items assembled in a way that allowed the food to be conveniently served and allowed us to make out plates according to our own personal desires. I have now placed her as my go to option when I am ever in need of her services!"* ~ **Kiera Stafford**

**December 2, 2019**

"*Those vegan treats were amazing. I ate them today*"! ~ **JaMar Elliott**

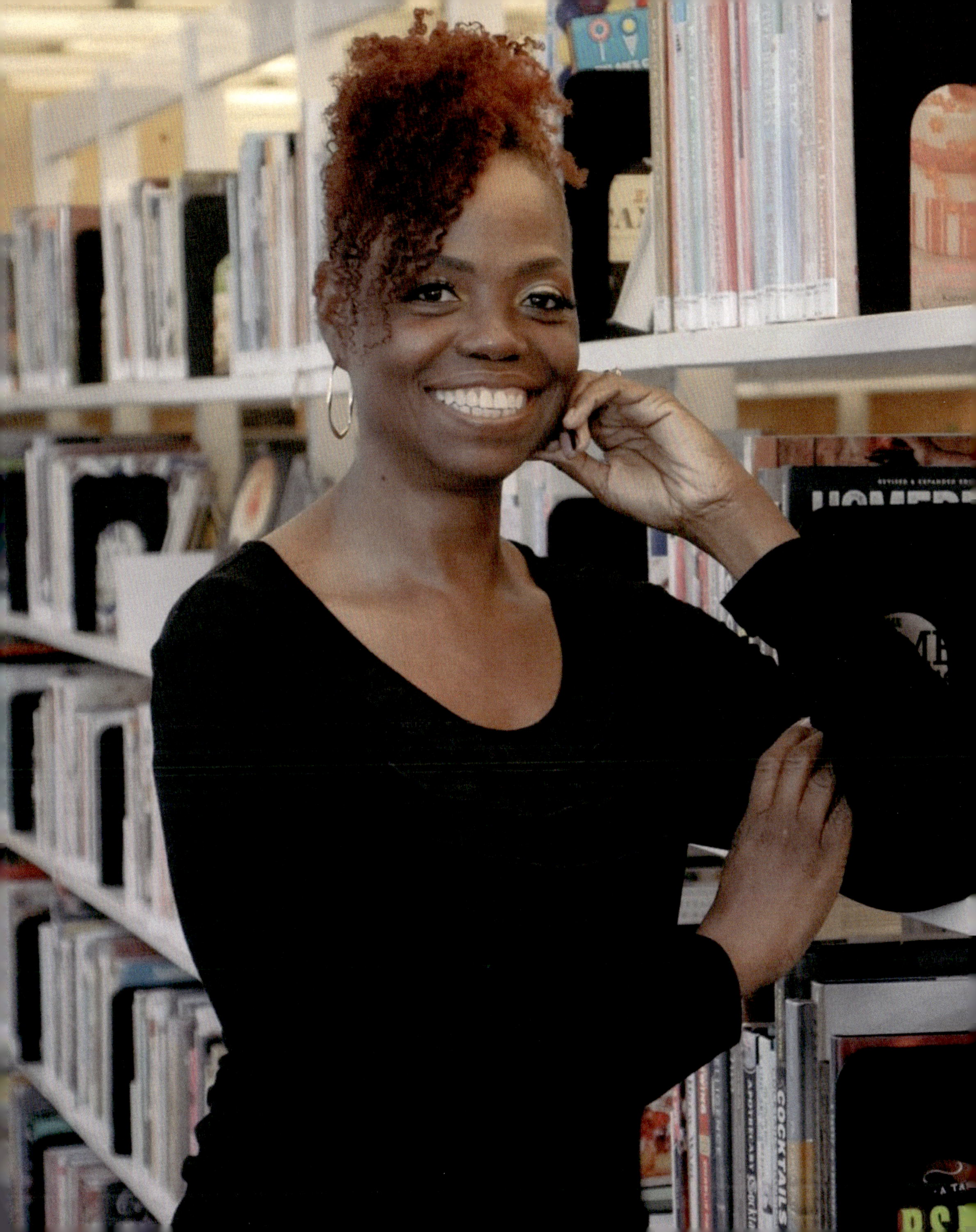
COCKTAILS

**About the Author**

Felisa transitioned cold-turkey to a vegan/plant-based lifestyle because she decided to no longer take her health for granted.

As a Transformational/Lifestyle Health Coach, She not only shares her personal vegan journey, but as a Vegan/Plant-based Transformational Coach she also uses her platform to help others. Felisa wants to inspire, encourage, and provide a level of accountability that she feels is currently absent and missing in the healthy living environment. She has earned her M.A. in Family Life Education Studies. Her \knowledge, experience, and expertise; along with a keen desire to share delicious and flavorful vegan recipes have a positive impact on her clients. Whether you are vegan or plant-based, or just looking to incorporate an abundance of fresh fruit and vegetables into your diet, Felisa is helping people lead more compassionate thriving lives!

**Felisa Cargile, M.A., Poet, Transformational/Lifestyle Health Coach**

Made in United States
Orlando, FL
04 November 2026

90201278R00081